STRESS OUT!

for Cats, Dogs & their People

STRESS OUT!

for Cats, Dogs & their People

Sumner M. Davenport

introducing co-authors
Janine Allen
Ellen Bishop
Dr. Kim Bloomer
Tammy Lawrence-Cymbalisty
Dina Discola
Lynda Fishman
Eileen Gould
Sue Heldenbrand
Victoria Loveland-Coen
Sally Shields
Dr. Joy Vanderbeck

Self-Investment Publishing © 2012

STRESS OUT FOR CATS, DOGS AND THEIR PEOPLE.

Sumner M. Davenport, also introducing co-authors and other contributors

"How Much is that Doggie in the Window", "A Charlie Brown Christmas" ©Dina Discola; "I Rescued a Human Today" Janine Allen ; "A Puppy Mill Mom", "My House", "Charlie", "Rhettung", "Shelter Vet", Foster Parents", Rescues", ©Ellen Bishop; "My Wife's Cat", © Bernard J.; "My Running Partner", ©Victoria Loveland-Coen; "Shadrach the Teacher Dog", Shadrach the Neo Mastiff ...nuthin' but the dog in him!" ©2009 Kim Bloomer, V.N.D. Used with permission from the book Animals Taught Me That.". First published by Crossbooks 11/16/2009; "Cat's and Children", ©Sally Shields; "If I Knew Then What I know Now", ©Marcia Klark.; "Live Life More Like A Dog", ©Eileen Gould. "Only My Dog", ©Katie W.; "The Message in Poop",
©Leslie May; "Natural Healing", ©Sue Heldenbrand; "Jades Halloween Adventure", ©Bridget Clovis "To Leash or Not to Leash", ©Mike Branson; "Dog Parks", © Sharone Ray; "Car Rides", ©Cindy S.; "Miracles Last Miracle", ©Dr. Joy Vanderbeck.; "Making a Difference", ©Lynda Fishman. All other book content ©2009, @2012 Self Investment Publishing and Sumner M. Davenport. All rights reserved.

Self Investment Publishing
2219 E. Thousand Oaks Blvd. Suite 102-386
Thousand Oaks, CA 91362

Graphics, Michael Lewiston, Michele Stuart
Research & Editing, Sumner M. Davenport
Copy Editor, Marge Diehl

Published by Self Investment Publishing ©2012

10 9 8 7 6 5 4 3 2 1

ISBN 10: 0-9815238-7-0
ISBN 13: 978-0-9815238-7-3

Other Books by Sumner M. Davenport:
Stress Out, show stress who's the boss
It works with Simple Keys
How to Turn your Ideals and Desires Into Reality
The "G: spot, the ecstasy of life through GRATITUDE
Insight & Discovery
The Magic Story
No More Damaged Goods
Solve the Entrepreneur Puzzle
The Difference a Day Makes
The Best and Last Self Help Book You Will Ever Need
Co-author in The Speakers Anthology

Introducing co-authors and other contributors:
Co-author bio's in the Authors Section at the back of book.

Janine Allen
Ellen Bishop
Dr. Kim Bloomer
Mike Branson
Bridget Clovis
Tammy Lawrence- Cymbalisty
Marge Diehl
Dina Discola
Lynda Fishman
Eileen Gould
Sue Heldenbrand
Bernard J.
Marcia K.
Victoria Loveland-Coen
Sharone Ray
Cindy S.
Sally Shields
Dr. Joy Vanderbeck

TABLE OF CONTENTS

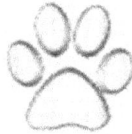

DEDICATION

To all the beautiful angels in fur
that have blessed our lives
and who have attempted
to teach us unconditional love.

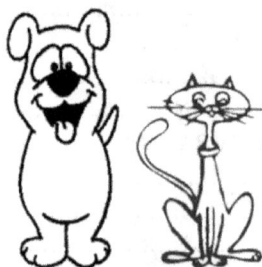

INTRODUCTION

*"If animals could speak the dog
would be a blundering outspoken fellow,
but the cat would have the rare grace
of never saying a word too much."*
~ Mark Twain

The intention of this book is to raise awareness, educate and inspire, and to assist in raising well needed funds for animal charities and their support groups.

You may be familiar with several celebrities who champion for the welfare of animals, such as Betty White, Ellen DeGeneres, David Bromstad, Sandra Bullock, Pauley Perrette, Selena Gomez and others. At the same time, many everyday people are just as committed and active in their support of adopting and proper care our animal companions. You will meet a few of them in this book.

Domesticated animals, especially cats and dogs, have been companions in our lives and homes for thousands of years. The American Association of Human-Animal Bond Veterinarians (AAH-ABV) defines the bond that people have with their animal companions in part as, "The human-animal bond is a mutually beneficial and dynamic relationship between people and other animals."

According to Scientific American, the domestic house cat is the most popular animal companion in the world. (Of course, dogs would have a bark about that.) A third of American households have feline members, and more than 600 million cats live among humans worldwide. On the farm, cats are vital to rodent and bird control in grain, seed and gardening areas. When people began inviting cats into their homes, they used ashes, leaves and plain sand as early litter box fillers. When clay litter was introduced in 1947, cats became even more welcomed in people's homes and families.

Throughout history and still today in some rural areas, dogs are used to assist with the livestock. Many people rely on their dogs for an early warning system, as well as protection against intruders both human and animal.

The animal-human bond is a most beautiful lifelong relationship. We bond with our cats and dogs in a number of ways: by showing how we love them, playing with them, giving them special treats and taking steps to minimize their stress and anxiety. In return we receive unconditional love, devotion and several health benefits including reduction of our own stress. Research has indicated that interaction with animal companions can assist to relieve human stress. One study reported at the American Heart Association Scientific Sessions, showed that a few minutes with a dog before an upcoming surgical operation, patients have experienced a 37% reduction in their anxiety levels.

During my research for this book, I met several people who didn't know that cats and dogs could be stressed. Dogs that are stressed out can develop certain stress behaviors such as pacing, whining, barking, chewing and in some cases self-mutilation. Some of the ways we treat our animals adds to their stress, and to our own. When people leave their home for a few hours or days, many will think about a dog sitter or boarding place. Many times cats are simply left alone with the thought that they are less maintenance, and need no daily care. Cats left alone can suffer from separation anxiety or loneliness, which can lead to destructive behaviors to relieve their stress.

There are things we can do to reduce, avoid and eliminate many stressors for our animal companions and ourselves. They can be negatively affected by our attitudes, energy, environment and our caregiving. They depend on us, their people, to keep them safe and healthy.

Cats and dogs are our special companions, giving unconditional love. When they are kittens and puppies, these gentle beings steal our hearts with their cute faces and playfulness. Just like children, as they get older they change and require us to help them learn their boundaries, learn the best behaviors, eat right and so they can grow into the best they can be in our home. Anyone who shares a home with these adorable creatures knows that cats and dogs adopted humans as pets long ago, not the other way around. Lives are changed when you share love with an animal companion.

> *"Dogs believe they are human.*
> *Cats know they are Gods!"*
> ~Anonymous

Adopting a cat or dog is a LIFETIME commitment. Relinquishing an animal to the pound or abandoning an animal that was once a devoted companion in your family can be the end of their life - literally!

During the lifetime of your animal companion you may experience many life changes; such as moving to a new home, changing or losing your job, relationship transitions and other life events. In addition, you and/or your animal companion may have medical problems or other adjustments. Are you willing to commit to your companion, no matter what? If it doesn't work out or you change your mind, there is no such thing as kitty or doggie divorce and you both moves on to new partners. *One of you may not survive the breakup.* Our shelters and rescues are bursting at their seams. **Thousands of cats and dogs are euthanized every day** at animal shelters across the country because of the over population and the lack of funds to care for these discarded friends.

A friend sent me this heart-stopping quote: *The only difference between a human jail and most animal shelters: For a cat or dog, if someone doesn't bail you out in just a few days, it's mandatory execution... even though you are innocent.*

Before adopting your next cat or dog, ask yourself if you are committed to be in it for the long haul. Many can live 15 years or more. These days some relationships including marriages and careers don't last that long. These animal companions will love you for their lifetime, and they hope you will return the same love.

You hear it every day - people unwittingly refer to their animal companions as "just a dog" or "just a cat." Some people unfortunately believe that these little beings have little value and deserve little respect. True animal people know the difference they make in our lives, and the difference we can make in theirs. In this book, we use the words "animal companion", "guardian"; and "sharing your home with an animal," rather than "ownership" or "pet." Titles are powerful words. Guardian or companion has a different energy and feeling than being an owner of something.

This book is a collection of real life stories from people who have learned something about themselves through the cats and dogs in their care. They have also learned how to better care for their animal companions which can then reduce the stress for both. In these personal stories you might read something that helps you to understand your animal companion's stress, or find a way to prevent accidents, injury and some illnesses.

Contributor, Dr. Kim was motivated to increase her knowledge and expand her profession because of a large dog with an even larger heart. Dina learned the real value of a dog and found a place that needed the love she had to share. Tammy learned how animals experience loss and the need for closure. Michael found compassion in the most unexpected soft touch on his knee.

We hope to inspire you, educate you and provide solutions to some of your frustrations and questions. Not everyone shares the same opinions. Whereas one chapter author strongly opposes prescriptive drugs, another saw how the medication helped to heal her beloved companion. Keep an open mind, and see where you might learn something that will help you and your animal companions.

This book endorses adoption over purchase. We encourage you to visit the local shelter or online adoption sites first. You may be surprised to find that nearly every breed of cat and dog has a rescue organization. Many animals are waiting for their furrever home. Your perfect companions are waiting in these places for you.

Cat's ...
Just What Good
are They?

"The smallest feline is a masterpiece."

~ Leonardo da Vinci

There are so many good reasons to share your home with a cat. Cats can help to lower your stress. Playing with a cat can elevate levels of serotonin and dopamine, which calm and relax. It only takes 15 to 30 minutes with a cat to feel less anxious and less stressed.

Cats can help you heal faster. People with cat companions tend to be healthier, and go to the doctor less often than non-cat people. Some rehab facilities and hospitals employ "therapy cats", to assist sick people feel more connected and even heal faster.

Cats are good for the heart. Having a cat companion can reduce your risk of heart attack by thirty percent. A recent study by researchers at the University of Minnesota[1] found that feline-less people were at higher risk for cardiovascular disease than those with cat companions. Over the twenty years of one study, people who never shared their home with a cat were 40% more likely to die of a heart attack than those who had.

Cats are good to ward off strokes. People who live with cats have fewer strokes than people who don't. Researchers speculate that cats may have a more calming effect on their people than other animals do. Sitting and stroking a cat then becomes the focus of the person's interest. We can only hold one thought at time in our mind, so instead of worrying about something stressful - think how soft the cat's fur is, the soothing sound of their purr and the warmth they offer in your lap.

Cats are good for stretching. An article in Arthritis Today[2] advises people to take a cue from their cat companion. Watch how many times she stretches every day. Each time your cat stretches, attempt to mimic the same long body stretches. Stretch from side to side and stretch each limb. Although some cat positions may be difficult for a person to duplicate, it can be beneficial to follow the basic ones. Breathe deeply when stretching to also relax your mind and reduce the stress on your body.

Cats are good company. A UK study[3] revealed that cats helped their persons overcome feelings of loneliness. A majority sometimes preferred to share their feelings with their cat rather than a partner or friend. Cats can keep a secret. They don't judge us; they just love us. When I went through several rough bumps in my life, Lancelot heard it all and he kept my secrets. This study also showed that children regarded their cat as a close friend.

Cats are good for a good night's sleep. Cats are excellent snugglers. In this same UK study more than half of the participants revealed that they enjoyed a better night's sleep with their cat on the bed than they did with their partner in the bed. These same people also admitted that they would tolerate their cat taking most of the bed covers at night but not their partner doing that. Many people who share their beds with a cat will admit to the contortions they take to get out of bed without disturbing the cat. Only to find that once they are out of bed, their adorable friend is out of bed as well and usually right at their feet.

While we may ponder the many good reasons for cats they may be thinking, "**Meow. What good are these humans?** *They are so distracted all the time; they miss the beauty in the wee things floating all around them. They forget that their music comes from within. They overlook so many opportunities to see things from various perspectives. They miss the warmth of a sunbeam streaming through a window, and the chirping of fascinating activity all around them. They can be so frustrating, so self-involved....... wait, do I hear a can opener?*"

"Ever consider what they must think of us?
I mean, here we come back from a grocery store with the
most amazing haul of chicken, pork, half a cow.
They must think we're the greatest hunters on earth!"
~ Anne Tyler

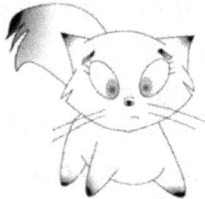

It's *Just* a Dog!

"He is your friend, your partner,

your defender, your dog.

You are his life, his love, his leader.

He will be yours, faithful and true,

to the last beat of his heart.

You owe it to him to be worthy of such devotion."

~ Original author unidentified ~

I asked some of my friends who share their lives with dogs, how they feel when someone says "he's *just* a dog". (Emphasis on *just*.)

Here are a few responses:

When someone says it's *just* a dog I wonder how much they truly care about their dog or any dogs and put them into a category of "*it's just*". Do they ever say , "It's *just* a child?"

Someone who says, "it's *just* a dog", has never allowed themselves to feel unconditional love.

Someone who says "it's *just* a dog" may not understand that dogs have feelings. On the contrary, dogs instinctively know when they are welcomed. They can have their hearts broken, just like people. You can see evidence of this is from visiting dogs in the shelter who've been abandoned or left behind. You can see dogs that cower, tails down, ears down when they hear their person ranting, scolding, and displaying anger - even when it is not directed at the dog. It's worse when it is directed at the dog.

Someone who says "it's *just* a dog" is someone who will abandon their dog or dump them at the shelter, because they are moving and are not willing to take the time to find a new home that is pet friendly.

Someone who says "it's *just* a dog" is someone who will feed their dog just anything and then be more angry than concerned when their dog is sick or hurt; acting as if it's the dog's fault.

Someone who says "it's *just* a dog" is someone who won't take the time to correctly train their dog, and yells at the dog or hits it when the dog does something wrong. These people don't take any responsibility for the things their dogs do because of the lack of proper training.

Someone who says "it's *just* a dog" is one who thinks that dog fighting should be legal sport.

Someone who says "it's *just* a dog" is one who thinks that spay/neuter is an inconvenience and all dogs should have as many puppies as people want them to have, without consideration as to what it does to the dog, the population or our shelters.

Someone who says "it's *just* a dog" is one who has never allowed themselves to feel the true companionship that a dog can provide.

Someone who says "it's *just* a dog" has never accepted that the fun of play with a dog that cannot be duplicated with any person. It is unique to the dog.

There's so many other ways that a person who says "it's *just* a dog" shows that they have either a limited understanding or limited love for a most amazing creature. These amazing animals can give sight to someone who's lost theirs; arms to someone who can no longer use theirs; companionship to the elderly in assisted living homes or someone who is home bound; protect and serve our military, police forces and communities by finding bombs and dangerous persons.

These amazing animals can find drugs, detect cancer, alert their humans of danger, find someone who is lost, and bring joy that cannot be measured.

The next time you hear yourself or someone say "it's *just* a dog". Ask - *"what exactly does that mean?"* You may learn something about yourself or someone else.

Regardless of the person's attitude, a dog may be thinking **"Arf. They're just a human**. *They only have two legs and can't run as fast as I can. They always seem to be in a hurry and miss many of the small joys in their path. They place conditions on love, and hold onto grudges that kill their spirit. They know the right things to do, and many times ignore the best solutions for their life. They limit how far they go. They forget how much can be heard without music or the TV blaring. They sit too long when they could be playing, or just visiting everything in nature. They forget how to share, and to let someone else have the stick from time to time. I believe that they do the best they can, but they sometimes forget that I am more than just a dog."*

"Outside of a dog, a book is probably man's best friend;

inside of a dog, it's too dark to read."

~ Groucho Marx

SAVING LIVES

"Anyone who thinks that money can't buy happiness
has never paid an adoption fee."

~ Original author unauthenticated

Almost daily, television ads are asking for help for rescued and abused animals. The voiceover also quotes statistics on how many animals are euthanized each week. We have recently witnessed on the news, police and animal services raids on homes where an overabundance of animals are being kept. These are not isolated cases.

Kitten and puppy mills and the stores that support them have also been in the news more consistently for the past few years. They bring attention to the heartless conditions the "breeder' animals endure, and how these litters are showing up with health conditions and behavior problems due to over breeding, lack of proper prenatal care and lack of proper health treatment or feeding. With research and tenacious rechecking, you may find some responsible and ethical breeders who are in the business because of the love they have for that specific breed. These breeders know that pregnancy and birth is taxing on the body so they limit the number of litters their cats and dogs will have. They raise the kittens and puppies in a loving environment, take care to safeguard their health and they carefully screen any prospective purchasers. Many of them contractually require that their litters be spayed/neutered in an attempt to protect the breed. Pet stores that sell cats and dogs appear to be making more effort to assure their customers that their animals come from reputable breeders, however as you will read in Dina's story, "How Much Is That Doggie In the Window?" even with "papers" she later discovered that her dog's "breeder" was investigated several times for being a puppy mill.

Although it appears that fewer retail stores are selling cats and dogs, there are still an uncontrolled number of backyard and non-reputable breeders. Several times a year we see people outside of shopping malls and on street corners with the little ones in a box and selling them to anyone with the requested dollars. Some states have enacted laws against sidewalk sales of animals, however, these little ones can melt a heart and cause a hasty purchase. There is no way to know how many of these innocent little ones are going to a loving furrever home, and which ones will be abused or later abandoned because they had medical problems because of their unhealthy birthplace.

Regardless of the breed of cat or dog you are looking for, there is most likely a rescue organization for that breed. They myth I hear most often is that shelter cats and dogs have something wrong with them, and that's why they're in a shelter. Some of these precious beings in the shelters may have been rescued from the street and may have developed a few medical conditions because of the harsh conditions they were subjected to in order to survive. Many others are abandoned or relinquished by their people who no longer want to care for them or made a decision that something or someone else was more important than the commitment they originally made to the animal. There are some animals taken to the shelter or local pound because their human wasn't physically or mentally capable of being able to continue to give them the best quality of life.

Most of us have no problem buying a used car or borrowing a friend's used clothing; but for some reason we erroneously think that the shelter and rescue dogs are "used", less valuable and problematic. This couldn't be farther from the truth. The only thing these animals did was being born at the wrong place. They may have trusted a person who then gave up on them; someone who decided the new home or new relationship was more important; or just used one of a few other irresponsible excuses for changing the course of this animal's life. In my volunteer work at a local shelter, I saw cats and dogs of all ages and breeds come through those doors. Some were assessed to be pedigreed. Many of these warm hearts could have been adopted if someone had started at the shelter first when looking for their special companion.

Laws have been passed in some states that retail stores can no longer sell commercially bred animals. In southern California two of the largest retail pet stores, PetCo and PetSmart have ceased selling cats and dogs they once obtained from breeders. Instead, they host special adoption days at their stores to showcase animals from the local shelters. Other smaller licensed pet stores are beginning to do the same.

Just like people there is no guaranteeing that a cat or dog will be in perfect health and behavior during their entire life, including those purchased from a breeder. Love and patience is involved. The right one, however, will be perfect for you and your home.

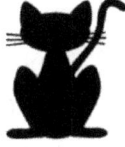

Top Reasons to Adopt a Black Cat

🐾 Black goes with everything. Black cats will match any decor.

🐾 Black is very slimming. Holding a black cat will make you appear slimmer.

🐾 Black is always are always sleek, stylish and elegant looking.

🐾 A lint brush isn't required for black-tie affairs.

🐾 They don't care what color you are.

🐾 In many cultures, Black cats can bring you good luck.

🐾 Black cats are the least likely to be adopted.

🐾 You will same them from those who want to torture them at Halloween.

🐾 **Best reason:** You will save their life
and they will return the love

*"A black cat crossing your path signifies
that the animal is going somewhere."*
~ Groucho Marx

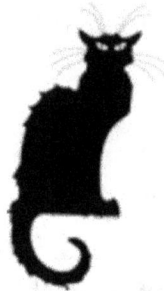

We Saved Each Other's Lives

"There is no psychiatrist in the world
like a dog licking your face."
~ Ben Ames Williams

I had no forewarning how a ten pound little dog could have such a large impact on my life. This little champion healed my heart in ways I could never imagine. I hadn't lived with dogs, since I was a teenager.

It started when a new neighbor moved in next door. It seemed that every night she was bringing home a different dog. I wasn't sure if she was trying them out and then returning them, like exchanging outfits at the mall, or if she was some sort of halfway house. It was, of course, more like the latter. She worked at a local shelter. From time to time, the animals who had been sheltered there the longest were allowed to have overnight visits with one of the staff. It was one way they hoped to minimize kennel stress. I was impressed when she shared with me about her job and what a difference they hoped they were making in the lives of these cats and dogs.

She invited me to an information day "just to see." That's all it took. Once I heard the facts about discarded animals and those hungry hearts waiting to share love, I was compelled to volunteer. Volunteers were required to buy a logo t-shirt to identify ourselves as volunteers anytime we were on site. I purchased six. I knew I would be in there often and it saved on having to do laundry every day.

It had only been a short time since the loss of my beloved Lancelot, so I hesitated to spend time with the cats, and instead found myself warmly welcomed and comfortable with the little dogs. The bigger dogs seemed more than I could handle, plus I still had some residual fear of dogs after being bit in the face as a child.

I was five years old and the time and I can still remember clearly hearing a voice seemingly in the distance saying "stay away from the dog" just as I reached him -- face to face. I was just tall enough so that my face was at the dog's mouth level. Then it was pain, blood and doctors; more pain and a lifetime memory that dogs cause pain and should be avoided. Years later my father stopped by the local dog pound on the way home from work and selected a beagle puppy as a playmate for us kids. My fear of dogs, however, was in place from my previous experience and I spent very little time with our new puppy, and even less after he grew up from his puppy size.

When I was a teenager my father had Australian shepherds as working dogs and companions. Even though I was around them as they worked and played, I was always on alert and never sat down at any time when I would have my face at their face level. Children who have had a painful or scary experience with an animal can carry that memory and fear for years, and sometimes their lifetime. I didn't want to be controlled by this fear, yet at the same time; I wasn't jumping at the chance to hug these dogs around their necks or body, as my father did. If they got on the couch next to me, I found another place to sit. These dogs never bite anyone that I saw. In fact, they were assigned the task of babysitting some of the younger children who came to visit from time to time. Being working dogs, these gentle beasts would round up children similar to the animals they were trained to corral. Gentle nudging, blocking paths and occasionally picking one up by the butt of the diaper. Even though the kids didn't always like being confined to a specific area of the yard, they loved the dogs and the dogs appeared to love the job.

Other than one friend's Golden Retriever, Mattie, and another friend's Collie blend, Honey, who both demanded to be my friend and exercised great patience until they won my trust, I have avoided big dogs. At the shelter it felt safer to work and play with the small dogs. Even though on the street I have met some seemingly vicious tiny dogs, they weren't as scary as my big dog memory from childhood. The small dogs at the shelter were all loving and playful. They appeared to be grateful for the attention and care.

When I started doing my volunteer time at the shelter and caring for the dogs, I soon discovered how much fun it was. It seem to fill a missing part in my life I hadn't been aware was missing. It was different than the void left by the departure of my cat, Lancelot. It was like a call back to something fun in my childhood. I could feel my stress ease with the wag of each tail and the happiness to see "me." Or the "me" at that moment.

Every few days I was at the shelter, playing toss and fetch, walking dogs and even cleaning kennels. There was a lot of expressed appreciation from the staff and even more from all the little dogs. If you want to feel useful and appreciated, this is the place.

Fortunately, many of the dogs were adopted quite quickly. No so for one type of dog. This is when I first learned about the "black dog syndrome." Some people have a preference for certain black dogs, i.e.: a black lab, however, for many people a black dog isn't even on their radar. Some say that it's because there isn't a contrast between the dark eyes and dark fur, so there's no emotional connection. Others perceive black dogs as somehow more aggressive or unfriendly. On the contrary, black dogs are not more aggressive than other colors of dogs. They can be very friendly and loving when living with a loving human companion.

I was introduced to Isaac, a ten pound MinPin/Chihuahua blend, with a shiny nearly all black coat. Only the smallest trace of white fur on his chest and under his chin. His dark eyes glistened whenever a person walked into his kennel and said hello to him. He was quiet and cautious. He had less interest in going outside to participate in toss and fetch with the other dogs, but preferred to sit on your lap and chew on his toy. Unfortunately, he had already been at the shelter for six months with no serious interest. It was heartbreaking to watch potential adopters walk by his kennel, without looking in, as if he didn't exist. He had been saved from death row at a county animal services shelter and brought to this no-kill shelter in hopes of giving him a furrever home and a new life. Because of his long time residence in this shelter he began to show signs of kennel stress. He would spin in one area, or pace across the short width of his kennel. When left alone, he would cower in the corner, with his ears down, and lowered eyes. You could hear his faint whining as he watched the people walk past his door. Kennel stress can be the end of the road for a dog at some shelters, but fortunately not at this shelter. For them it was a sign that something needs to be done fast, to get this dog into a home; even if it's a temporary foster home.

I was volunteering at the shelter that day, and had just left Isaac when the kennel manager approached me and asked if I would be willing to foster Isaac. I had never considered being a foster parent, didn't know what was required or even if I was capable of having a dog as my responsibility in my home. None of that came to mind when she asked if I would be willing to help Isaac, instead I heard myself say "of course I will" without hesitation. After lengthy instructions of what to do and not do, my car was loaded with a big dog crate, blankets, toys, food and a small dog, and I was on my way.

The first action he took after walking inside my home was to raise his leg and claim the plant by the door as his territory. Part of my responsibility as a foster mom was to train him to be potty trained and he had just shown me that we needed to work on that. Fortunately, I was familiar with Natures Miracle Odor Remover so no real harm was done to my plant or the floor.

It was an adjustment at first to have this little guy follow me all over the house. I was aware that I was always being watched. The next day I sent an email to the shelter telling them about our first night together and how funny it seemed to me to have a cute little guy find me so fascinating. It had been a long time since a handsome young man had watched me take a shower.

Even though Isaac was only ten pounds, and barely tall enough to reach my knees when standing on his hind legs, I could sense my old fear. Even little dogs can bite, so initially I was cautious around him. Two of the rules for a foster home, were to keep him off the furniture and he must sleep in a crate at night. If his furrever home wanted him on the furniture or their bed, they could allow it. It's easier to give permission than to take it away. As for sleeping in his crate, this kept a distance between us to help keep him from getting attached to me.

It didn't take long for this little guy to own real estate in my heart. He came to my home for a reason and I believe he knew right away that this was his furrever home. A big note here is that foster families are NOT obligated or even expected to adopt. In my case it was meant to be. I am considered a foster failure; however, that's one failure I don't mind.

Once he was legally a member of my family, I renamed him to Tigger. Like the character in Winnie the Poo. He is always very happy. When he knows it's time for a walk, he bounces and bounces until the harness is on. One time, when I bent down too soon to leash him, my cheekbone got the top of his head on one of his bounces and I ended up with a black eye. I love his enthusiasm, however, I'm now trained to ask him to sit and wait for him to obey. Then when bending down to leash him I continue to be mindful by guarding my face for that potential rogue bounce.

Tigger came into my life at the perfect time. My schedule immediately changed. It had been a while since my last marathon, and my exercise routine had become more than just lax, it was almost nonexistent. On most days, I am fortunate to have a 30 second commute to my desk. That also means I have to schedule myself to get away from the desk and do a little exercise. Prior to Tigger coming to live with me, there were many days I would sit at my desk, and then discover that hours had passed and I hadn't gotten up from my chair. Having him in my home needing incremental walks took away some of my "not right now" excuses. Working on the housetraining with him, with walking him every few hours, I was also giving myself necessary breaks. A few times a week we walk at the local park, so we both have the benefit of smelling fresh cut grass, feeling the soft breezes, see the rustling trees and hearing the birds sing. Our outside time became walking meditations for both of us.

Tigger helps my schedule throughout the day as well. He has one dog bed next to my desk where after his breakfast he takes the first of his many naps. It's cute to hear those doggie dream noises while I work. The sound always brings a smile to my face, and I have to control myself not to interrupt his nap admiring his cuteness by crawling over to get a closer look.

He always wakes up happy, something we can all learn from our dogs. He is ready for what's next in his day, which may simply be the same as before he went to sleep or the same as yesterday, but he wakes with an excitement for the adventure. When he wants my attention he "noses me." Tigger is not a licking dog, so instead he bumps me with his nose. That can be a real attention getter when that cold wet nose hits my warm leg.

I am also fortunate that Tigger is not a barking dog - well.... - unless there are dogs on television. We watches television together, with him snuggled between me and a couch pillow, usually slobbering on one of his chew bones. All is well until he sees a dog on the screen. I can't figure out if he thinks the dog is coming into his home or what?? It's something I've worked on with him. My objective is to train him that dogs on television are a good thing, and sometimes come with scratches behind his ears or a special treat. The shelter where he used to reside encouraged positive reinforcement training. They recommended specific books and television shows to assist me in learning so I could better train him. I've learned positive reinforcement training from watching a dog trainer on the Animal Planet channel. When I'm watching a show with dogs, or a dog commercial comes on, I either give him scratches behind his ears or give him a treat while repeating he is a good dog. This show explained that this type of training method can train the dog to see that what they used to bark at or aggress towards, is really something that they can enjoy or feel is good for them. If when they see this perceived threat they are getting something pleasant or tasty, the good is reinforced.

I have been accused of being overly protective of Tigger however; he depends on me for his safety and well-being. He is a companion who is happy to see me every time I walk in the room. He shows me affection by wagging his tail and bouncing with joy when I talk to him. He gives me another happy reason to get up in the morning. Because of him, we have met some other nice dogs and their interesting people at the park.

It didn't take very long for him to be housetrained. He now sits and stays on command (for a while, anyway. We're still working on this.) It was important to train him to wait at the front door and not go through until he received the okay command from me.   This keeps him from dashing to, or through the door when it opens into the street or the pathway of people and other animals. He waits for the command while I assess who is outside and what other dogs might be there, both on and off leash.   When I say OK, he then follows me through the door.

When he sees me preparing myself for bed in the evening, he puts himself to bed, either in his own bed or on his side of my bed, He now walks with a gentle leash and he waits at corners for my command when it is safe for us to cross. We don't know why he was dumped at the pound, but it was his lucky day when the shelter folks rescued him before he met a terrible fate there.

Now I have a yoga partner living with me who does an authentic downward dog; an exercise partner, a playmate and a walking meditation companion. He adds joy to my days and laughter simply watching him and Merlin rough and tumble. (Read about Merlin in the story chapter, *"An Unexpected*

Addition to the Family.") I still can't understand the black dog syndrome and the "not being able to connect to the eyes" excuse. When I look at his cute face, I see the glimmer in two beautiful eyes that can see directly into my soul. My old fear of dogs is not even a faint thought around Tigger. He is so cute and lovable; I can't stop myself from hugging him and kissing his forehead. Yes, sometimes he loses patience with me and he growls. Doesn't bother me a bit. My face so close to his and all I feel is joy.

"Sophie, my dog, is the high
in the highlights of my life."

~ Lauren Bacall

How Much is That Doggie in the Window?

By Dina Discola

Hundreds of potential dog owners ask this question every day. I asked this question in 2002 when I saw a four month old blue and white Italian Greyhound at pet store. I went in every day for a week to visit him and then considered making the purchase. He was so beautiful and seemed so lonely sitting in his cage. When I pet him, I felt as if I was petting the dolphin I had met in Hawaii many years ago. There was hardly any fur but he was soft to the touch. When I took him out of his cage, he would nuzzle his nose right into the corner of my neck. He was perfect! I couldn't stop thinking about him.

The owners actually knew my father and said that they would give me a "deal" on him as he was getting too big. He was originally $1099 + tax but they gave him to me for a total of $838.93. Even though they said this was a "deal", I still thought it was very expensive but I bought him anyway.

I named him Georgio for a few reasons: he was a very curious puppy and reminded me of the character Curious George. My best friend is named after his father (George), and of course, I had to have something Italian in his name as I am 100% Italian and he is an Italian Greyhound, hence, Georgio Armani came to mind. So that was it!! Georgio was a fine name for such a cute little guy.

After his first year, Georgio started to lift his left leg every now and again. I didn't really think anything of it at the time, until a few years later when he started to lift it a lot. I asked my vet what he thought might be wrong and he said it looked like a luxated patella. I had no idea what this was and asked for his advice. He told me that if it got worse, Georgio would need surgery. At age 6, Georgio did undergo surgery for his luxated patella. When I went to pick him up, the surgeon said that the leg would heal just fine, but unfortunately, he saw evidence of "chronic bilateral tarsal ventral instability" and that eventually Georgio would lose the ability to walk in his back legs and they would slowly give out. He did not want to fix them now and he described the surgery as painful. He would have to do bone grafting and bone fusion and put pins and/or a plate in each of Georgio's legs. Recovery would take anywhere between six weeks to three months and he would need to be confined. The cost of this surgery would range between $5400-$8000 depending on the surgeon I chose. The first surgery was approximately $3500. Two years later, Georgio was walking on his shins and his bones. He was starting to wear through his skin which eventually got to the bare bone and he started to bleed. I had a consultation and scheduled the surgery. I spent almost $10,000 on the two surgeries when all was said and done.

The reason I have told this story is because I am convinced that Georgio is a victim of a puppy mill! I have to admit that if I knew then what I know now, things would have been a lot different. First, I would have rescued a dog and not purchased one from a pet store. I would have educated myself on where dogs come from that end up in pet stores and have a good and clear understanding of what puppy mills are. When the pet store gave me Giorgio's paperwork, they handed me his "papers". One of the papers almost looked like a family tree. The paperwork had photos of his mother and father. On the left side, it said the breed: (IG), color: blue and white and the breeder's name. Now that I see this, my stomach turns inside out, but back then, I had no idea what this meant. After I did some research, I found out that this "breeder" had numerous USDA violations a couple of years prior to my purchasing Georgio. It was reported that this breeder had 976 adult dogs and 534 puppies on their property. When I had asked the owners of the pet store for information about where Georgio came from, they stood behind this breeder.

After watching Georgio's condition begin to deteriorate, I called the pet store and spoke with the owner. I told him about Georgio and how much money I would be spending. This type of physical problem he was now suffering from, can be seen most often in puppy mill dogs. I wanted to give the store owner an opportunity to do the right thing and at least help with some of the expenses. His only response was that the breeder where Georgio came from is no longer in business and that Georgio is too old now and because of this, he cannot help. I explained that blood work on Georgio is 100% fine, however, it is all the issues with his joints, bones that have been affected which is a correlation to his breeding. In fact, I explained that after doing further research on this breeder, I read about other dogs who had hernia repair, mites, luxating patellas, kennel cough, behavioral problems, sneezing and giardia. After even further research, I found out that this breeder is not out of business. She is still located in the same place and is the main breeder and provider for a well-known large pet store chain who has investigated for dealing with puppy mills. I actually called this pet store and they confirmed that they get most of their dogs from this breeder and they claim on their website that they have been working with her since 1994. They also show a list of over 42 different breeds and claim that they usually carry these breeds throughout the year. The point I am making here is that I was lied to by the pet store where I purchased Georgio and people like this breeder, even after many violations, appears to continue to prosper in this horrible business of farming and brokering puppies.

The opportunity I have now is to spread the word on what I know regarding puppy mills and on adopting or fostering a rescue dog. Millions of people buy dogs from puppy mills each year, and most believe they are getting a dog from a "responsible" breeder. Irresponsible breeders and puppy mill owners count on people falling in love with their puppies, either in the pet store or through adorable photos on the internet. Also, people buy on impulse and emotion. You must know the facts first and do your homework. The statistics are astounding: about four million dogs are bred in puppy mills each year while nearly five million animals are killed in shelters each year and the numbers continue to grow. More than 20% of dogs in shelters are purebred. I have found that it is easy to find a rescued puppy or dog by visiting some websites or your local shelter.

You see, a few years back, I became a volunteer for a no-kill animal shelter and educated myself on how important it is to rescue or foster. There are so many animals that are in need of a good home if only people will take the time to educate themselves. I also took the time to learn about a therapy program and became a Certified Handler. In addition, I adopted a dog last year who almost lost his life due to kennel cough. His name is Charlie Brown (Read about him in the chapter *"A Charlie Brown Christmas"*) and he is a happy and healthy Boston Terrier. I found him through the bostonbuddies.org website. I saved Charlie's life. Now Georgio has a new brother and they are best friends. Although I wasn't educated years ago about pet stores and puppy mills, I now have followed-up, done my homework and have made lemonade out of a situation of lemons. I cannot change the past but I can make a difference now and in the future.

See "About the Authors" section to learn more about Dina Discola.

You can say any foolish thing to a dog,
and the dog will give you a look that says,
"My God, you're right! I never would've thought of that!"
~ Dave Barry

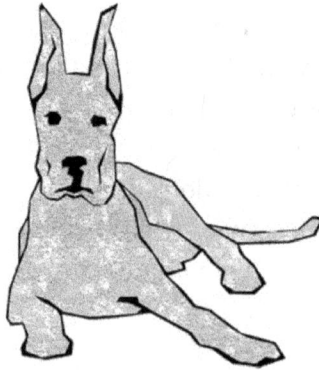

A Puppy Mill Mom

By Ellen Bishop

I've spent my life in a two by three box
Wire all around me, the doors have locks
My hair is matted, my feet are flat.
I've never known love, not even a pat.
My eyes are dim, my belly is round,
My callous pads have never touched ground.
I sleep in my urine and feces at night,
Squinting my eyes in morning's bright light
Food and water they give me are old and stale.
This prison I live in is worse than a jail.
My life is a breeder in some puppy mill
The back woods of nowhere up on a hill.
I don't see a vet and haven't had shots.
My captors are cruel keeping me in a box.
My litters of puppies born all in a row.
What happens to them, I'll never know.
They are taken from me at one month old,
Off to some pet store they are sold,
Just to provide for some persons greed,
Without one thought to what comes of me.

Puppy mills are as inhumane as a fighting ring. The entire reason for the ownership of these animals is for the profit of a greedy person willfully neglecting the dogs in their care for the profit of their pockets. The animals are kept in horrendous conditions. The females are kept in tiny cages which are not cleaned. They are usually not provided with vaccinations, de-wormed, or groomed. The males are confined with them when they are in heat. Once the breeding has occurred, the males are then removed and placed into a separate room. They live in their own waste and birth happens under these same conditions. Their young are taken away as early as three weeks of age and sold to unsuspecting buyers. Some of these moms have been living this way for so long that they are untrusting of people. The only time they have even seen people was for food occasionally thrown to them and water given through the cage. One of our puppy mill moms, Cotton, came to us from just such conditions. She would try to bite anyone who opened her kennel door and had to be sent outside with protection from a garbage can lid to even place food in her dishes. Poor Cotton was a cockapoo and from the condition of her coat had never known a bath or brush. She was pregnant when seized by animal control and brought to us. After a few weeks, she stopped trying to bite us and would just hide her head in a corner when we approached. We knew she had to be close to delivery but feared she would not allow us near her pups when they arrived. Vigilantly, we continued to attempt to coax her into realizing that we were not there to harm her, but help. We tried treats, including cheese and hot dogs, to lure her near us. She insisted on keeping her head buried in the corner away from us.

On the day her litter arrived, we saw a small but promising change in Cotton. She was still leery of us but would allow us into her kennel to handle and check her puppies. This was the point we decided to find her a foster home. A wonderful lady stepped forward to care for Cotton. After four days, we released Cotton into her care, hoping she would progress further. As the pups grew, she became more open to the foster mom. Eventually, Cotton would be adopted by her foster mom and the pups adopted into wonderful families. She still fears new people but eventually comes around crawling on her belly to garner the attention offered. Her mom thinks she will never completely trust anyone after the years she spent as a puppy mill breeder but loves her and Cotton will spend the rest of her days with love and compassion, understanding that never again will she be subjected to the cruelty of her previous life.

See "About the Authors" section to learn more about Ellen Bishop.

"An animal's eyes have the power

to speak a great language."

~ Martin Buber

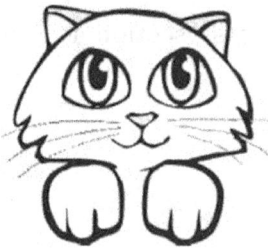

An Unexpected Addition to the Family

I've always been an animal lover. For most of my adult life, I have had cats in my home. Some of these went to other furrever homes, but Lancelot was my devoted cat companion for thirteen years. He was a beautiful short haired pure white cat with pink skin and one blue eye and one gold eye. Quite the looker! He traveled the world with me, including to houses when I sat with their animal companions while they traveled. He got along with everyone. He taught a few dogs that cats are not toys. I lost my devoted friend to cancer a few years ago. He left a void that has been difficult to fill.

To get my cat fix, I was spending time at a local rescue socializing and tending to the cats and kittens. Since I didn't think I was ready to adopt another cat, I fostered and then later adopted an adorable little dog. *(See story "We Saved Each Other's Lives")*

One late night while Tigger and I were taking our last walk before bedtime, something light colored and fuzzy jumped down from a tree and darted over to us. We have squirrels in our trees, so Tigger and I weren't startled, only curious. It turned out to be a very dirty kitten. He came directly to us, sat down and leaned up against Tigger's chest and purred. Almost like saying, *thank you for coming, please help me.* Tigger looked up at me over his shoulder as if to say "*can we keep him?*" Notice how well I hear animal speak.

Coyotes have been seen fairly regularly in our neighborhood recently, so this little guy was lucky to still be alive. Even though he was dirty, he was still light colored and easily seen in the moonlight. He could have been a small treat for a quick and hungry coyote.

Fortunately, my neighbor has three beautiful tuxedo cats and she had extra feline necessities to spare. Even at that late hour she responded to help the needs of this little guy. We made a place for him with small litter box and cat bed in one of my bathrooms. He didn't seem interested in food or water, and instead fell to sleep in my hands when I was wiping him off with a damp cloth. He appeared to be injury and pest free, just quite thin and tired.

I placed him in the little pet bed and he soon fell fast asleep with a loud purr. He didn't even seem to notice Tigger anymore; or us leaving the room so he could have privacy and safety during the night. It's been a while since I've had a kitten in my home, so fortunately my neighbor helped me determine how much food to give this little one this morning. The kitten gobbled up food faster than Tigger.

On our first walk the next morning, I placed signs with my phone number so the kitten could be returned to his rightful home if the caller could describe him. No one did. This was bittersweet. Later I took him to the vet for a full check up and make sure he was ok. The vet said he was about four months old and looked as if he had been on the street for a while, but not long enough to turn feral. He had ear mites and scratches, so he was cleaned up, shaved a little and sent home with antibiotics and healing herbs.

I use a holistic vet, and she appreciated what happened the night this little guy came home with me. Since the departure of my beloved Lancelot, I have consistently kept a small white cat night light glowing. That night after putting kitty to bed, this night light burnt out. Was it Lancelot telling me it was time for another purr in my home? Was he telling me he knew I would protect this little one until his responsible person came forth? Did he send him to me to live here? I meditated and didn't get answers; only peace, a peace I haven't felt since Lancelot left.

Merlin is now a permanent member of this family. He and Tigger run, tussle and play together like lifelong good friends. It's difficult at times to tell which one is the dog and which one the cat.

As soon as he was old enough, I had him neutered. It was then that I learned he was a flame point Siamese which explains why he doesn't seem to shed. Lancelot had left his white fur everywhere in my home, and on everything I wore. So he actually did go everywhere with me.

Nothing is safe from the speed of active small animals racing around the house, over and around furniture. Many friends told me that after Merlin was sterilized, he would become calmer without his testosterone. I guess no one told him that.

I've had to do some redecorating for his safety and my sanity. It's fun to witness.

I still miss my Lancelot; however, these two little fellows have brought so much love and laughter back into my home that was missing for a long while.

"Way down deep,

we're all motivated by the same urges.

Cats have the courage to live by them."

~ Jim Davis

Shadrach the Neo Mastiff ... nuthin' but the dog in him!

By Kim Bloomer, VND

In the late fall of 1999, we were still dog-less. Since Fridge had died, we'd not had the heart to try and find another dog, but he had been gone since January and I was beginning to have a major "fur withdrawal".

A very tragic incident was about to bring not only a new dog into my life, but also a dog that would turn my world upside down and send me on the path I believe God had always intended for my life. Shortly after Thanksgiving, I lost a very dear relative to a tragic death, and to this day it is extremely difficult to relive those memories. Friends and family members came from near and far to attend the funeral, and the next day a group of us joined together for a family outing and lunch. At one point during the afternoon one of my aunts happened to mention a dog which one of my cousins was hoping to give away to a good home. She already had too many dogs and simply could not afford to keep this very large and very needy puppy any longer. She had rescued him from a bad situation in which he had been neglected and was being left to die of starvation.

I asked my aunt, "What kind of dog is he?" and to my delight she answered, "He's some kind of Mastiff - a blue-colored one (blue brindle). That's all I know about him." All I heard was "MASTIFF" and "male" – exactly what I had had in mind! The very next week (it was the week before Christmas) we drove to my cousin's house in a nearby town to see him. She had told me he was a Neapolitan Mastiff , and during the entire previous week I had read everything I could find about the breed. I had also been buying all the required trappings for a dog; with the exception of his leash, I couldn't bear to use Fridge's things for another dog, so I needed a collar, training collar, dishes, food, treats, etc. It was an exciting time, but I was also nervous since I'd never owned a rescue dog with "baggage" before.

When we pulled up to my cousin's house all I saw was a VERY skinny, but cute in an ugly duckling sort of way, puppy out in the dog pen, barking furiously at us. Donnie only said, "Oh yeah, we're taking him!" but I wasn't so sure. My two previous dogs had been Golden Retrievers, and Neo's could not be a more different dog in every respect. I was horrified when I saw him; in fact, when I had first seen the pictures of the show dogs of the breed, I thought they looked like gargoyles. On closer inspection, all I saw in this puppy, whose name was "Shadow", was a skinny, raggedy, smelly little boy, but Donnie really wanted him and I couldn't bear the thought of just leaving him there and not knowing where and with whom he would end up. It was obvious he was VERY hungry too, because when he was brought in, the first thing he did was to try and "surf " the countertops in my cousin's kitchen. She had not fed him that day, fearing he would get carsick when he traveled with us, and I was very glad about that! I told her I'd feed him as soon as we arrived home.

Fortunately I had brought a little bag of treats with us, so on the forty-five minute drive home I gave him a few. He "sucked them up like a Hoover Deluxe", as Donnie always says. On the trip home I sat in the back seat with him and just held him close. I wanted to reassure him that there was nothing for him to fear. He didn't seem to be interested in us in the least, but only in whatever food we might have for him. When we finally got home I immediately put him on leash and walked him around the front yard, then took him in and let him walk around the house as well, still on lead. I showed him where his bed and food dishes were, and then I took him to the back yard and unleashed him so he could go potty. I noticed that his pee was an orange color instead of yellow - not a good sign; because of his severe starvation I've no doubt he had some kidney and liver damage.

Our first mistake was to feed him a large meal. You see, because of his starvation his body wasn't used to that much food at one time and was not in good enough shape to be able to assimilate all that we gave him. What went in came right out in pile after pile of poop – in the yard, not the house, thank God! He only had one accident in the house.

I believe that first day I must have picked up about twenty piles of poop, but the worst was yet to come. The most difficult part of bringing home a new dog, especially a puppy, is how they get through the dark of night. Shadrach's first night was absolutely horrible. At least I had given him a bath before that first day was over, but it didn't do much to improve his odor, because it was coming from inside him. I can only surmise that Shadrach had an incredible will to live and did so in spite of all the odds against him.

Before I proceed further with Shadrach's story, let me say that his now name comes from the Book of Daniel in the Bible. Three Jewish princes were thrown into a horrific fiery furnace because they refused to deny God, and they survived because the pre-incarnate Lord Jesus was with them. They came through the fire unscathed and their witness was an incredible testimony to everyone at the time, and it still is. The name just came to me, and I truly believe that the name "Shadrach" was the one God intended for him. Shadrach had experienced extreme abuse and neglect from the very beginning of his short life thus far, and yet he had survived "the fire". His former name, Shadow, certainly didn't suite his strong personality – not that he initially showed us any personality. Often when animals have suffered an abusive situation and are rescued from it they are renamed in order to give them a new beginning in every way, and that is exactly what we did with Shadrach.

We had borrowed a dog crate from a good friend for Shadrach to sleep in. It was a way to teach him where he was to sleep so that by the time he had outgrown the crate, he would automatically go to his own bed each night. However that first night in his new home had me doubting our decision to get another dog. He hollered and carried on as only a Neo Mastiff can - they are certainly one of the loudest and most vocal dogs I've ever encountered. During that long night I had visions of my golden retriever, Fridge, and how quiet he was, and the next morning the feeling that perhaps we'd made the wrong decision about him persisted. Donnie, however, told me later he intended to keep Shadrach no matter what I said.

I left him with Donnie, as I had promised I'd to go my young nephew's birthday party . I was so tired, and I wondered if I'd ever be in a quiet, peaceful place again. My selfish side had reared its ugly head for sure, and I hadn't even considered what a horrible go of things Shadrach had already endured. Now he was in an entirely new environment with new people and a better life ahead of him, and here I was complaining after only ONE day!

My neighbor's daughter soon came over to meet the new addition to our family. She is a fellow animal lover, and Shadrach took to her immediately. She was coddling that stinky guy in her lap and I just sat there looking at them, wondering how I could possibly have thought I was ready for a new dog. Poor Shadrach. I wasn't even giving him a chance. My friend and former vet tech who had loaned us the crate called to see how Shadrach was doing on his first day with us, and when I started to complain to her about his pooping, his smell, etc., she gave me one of the worst dressing downs I'd ever received – and it was well deserved too! She told me if I couldn't do the right thing by him, then the least I could do was find him a good "forever" home. I pondered all she said and the next morning, even with Shadrach's occasional hollering, I woke up and decided that we were going to run with it! I was ready to do everything in my power to see to it that Shadrach had a good home, with US! Donnie was ecstatic at my change of heart, and we agreed that together we would make it work.

I followed my friend's advice and started feeding Shadrach four small meals a day until his stomach was able to handle larger amounts and fewer meals – it didn't take rocket science to figure that one out, but apparently I needed to be reminded. To get Shadrach to go to bed at night and not be afraid of being locked in his kennel, I started singing to him – something only a dog could appreciate – and massaging him. The song I sang to him, I made up. To this day when I start singing it to him I can visibly see his body relax and any tenseness leave him. He'll even start wagging his tail when I sing it. Oh what we do for the ones we love.

On his second day, Shadrach was teaching me and we'd begun the amazing journey I had no idea we were going to take. Within a week he was eager to go to his "night nighty" (his crate) each night, and there was no more hollering throughout the night. One thing we did notice, however, was that occasionally he'd wake up startled from a nap or during the night and then begin a long, low, sorrowful howling. We'd rush to his bed or wherever he was sleeping and soothe him with a gentle touch. If it happened during the day he would sit up with a fearful look in his eyes and his heart would be hammering in his chest, almost as though he was having a nightmare. Only God and Shadrach knew what those "dreams" were all about – thankfully he hasn't had one of them in a very long time.

By Christmas Eve I felt confident enough that since he'd had a full week after coming to live with us to at least gain a little weight and adapt to his new life, he was ready for a walk in the park with me. When Shadrach saw Cora and Oreo, two of the dogs that were to become part of our regular morning dog play group, he actually appeared to skip, he was so excited to see other dogs again. As he was still a puppy, he was smaller than Cora the Aussie and Oreo the Labrador Retriever mix, so they were able to toss and tumble him all over the place. He reveled in the attention and fun. We had snow that first Christmas of our being together, and Donnie and I couldn't have been happier with the furry addition to our life. Shadrach completed our little family.

Most people pitied that poor little skinny boy the first time they saw him, but a few actually saw his tremendous potential. It wasn't long before Shadrach had put on weight, his coat gleamed, and the rascally look appeared in his eyes.

It was necessary for me to revise my entire workout routine. Since Shadrach slept in the weight room, I couldn't use it to lift weights before I went to the park as I had done previously. Instead I began going to the park earlier. I would walk him a couple of laps, put him in the car with a huge comforter, since it was still winter, and then run a few miles before taking him out of the car and off to his doggie play group. He practically dragged me around the park to reach the bridge leading to the "dog side" of the park, and everyone was amused by our "dog sled run" around the park, with me barely holding on for dear life. Shadrach was beginning to show great enthusiasm for everything he did.

The most difficult part of his rehab was to leave him alone for any length of time. I would run short errands only, trying to be away from home for no more than half an hour at a time, during which time I would put him outdoors so he'd not get into mischief or damage anything in the house. Once I tried leaving him in his crate, but as I drove up to the house I could hear him hollering and I knew that wasn't going to work. However, he still protested loudly when I left him outside as well.

Nevertheless, he eventually understood that I would return and he had nothing to be afraid of. When Donnie got home from work each night, I would turn Shadrach over to his care and say, "He's all yours. I'm done for." Shadrach was quite a handful, but actually no worse than any other puppy, the only difference being that he was a giant breed dog with a bit of baggage attached. Although he eventually grew to be larger than all his dog friends, he was still younger, and that was difficult for everyone to keep in mind.

When Shadrach was about six months old we took him to be neutered, something I would have certainly reconsidered if I knew then what I now know about animal health. Giant breed dogs should not be neutered before they are at least eighteen months to two years old since they need the hormones in order for their growth plates to fully close.
As Shadrach grew, so did our challenges with him. Mastiff s are a very independent- thinking, willful, stubborn breed of dog – they have to be, since their primary purpose is that of a

guardian. Once he came out of his shell, I had quite a character to contend with. He was no longer afraid of anything! Fortunately I had been doing basic command training with him, although he apparently still doesn't find any purpose in the "Come" command unless it's for food. I trained him from the beginning to not mouth or touch anything in the house; that was easy, since I simply replaced what I didn't want him to touch with something I didn't mind his touching, such as one of his own toys (which he has in abundance!)

We had our "yard challenges" as well. He thought hose nozzles and hoses were great fun to destroy, but we corrected that behavior right away by switching to metal nozzles and teaching him that the hose was off limits – except for summer time bathing which he loved as a puppy. Shadrach also thought digging up our nice lawn in the backyard was great fun. As soon as I caught him at it, I'd stop him with a firm "NO!" and then take him over to a portion of the yard reserved for his "digging", take hold of a paw and begin digging with it. I'd say, "Dig, dig, dig!" with a high-pitched tone of voice so he'd know that the intention was fun. He quickly got the message that it was okay to dig as much as he liked there, but not in the grass. When he had a "wild hair up his behind", such as dogs behave when excited, he'd run over to his "digging spot" and dig nearly to China! It was the funniest thing to watch.

It wasn't long before Shadrach outgrew his crate – his baby crib – and graduated to a big dog bed. He slept in his room without being locked in as he'd been conditioned to sleep in that spot. In fact, Shadrach outgrew everything – his collars, his bed, his toys, everything! He even outgrew ALL of his dog park buddies, with the group changing members on a regular basis. Shadrach remained the one constant at the park, as it was his favorite place to go. He has always loved interacting with fellow canines, although he has never enjoyed having them visit at our home.

Shadrach makes sure that we go for our daily walk, which helps us to stay healthy. He has made us aware of how important it is to eat food that is specific to our species. Shadrach has shown us that when we honor the laws of nature, which God instituted, we can be healthy and defy genetics. We both know that Shadrach was sent into our lives not because he needed saving but because we truly did. It was no accident that we were in need of a dog at the same time he was in need of a home. The road with Shadrach has never been easy, but he has been the best thing to happen to us! I feel as though he has shown me the path to full redemption for all my past mistakes. I am a better person because God sent a needy little puppy to a married couple in great need of life lessons that are often best learned through the love of an animal...a Neo Mastiff named Shadrach taught me all this and I'm still learning!

Read more about Shadrach in the chapter *"Shadrach the Teacher Dog"*. See "About the Authors" section to learn more about Dr. Kim Bloomer

A Charlie Brown Christmas

By Dina Discola

It was December, 2009 and I rescued my first dog, Charlie Brown.

I first read about Charlie on a Boston Terrier rescue website and his story broke my heart! At the time, my Boston (Oreo) was fourteen-years old and my Italian Greyhound, named Georgio, was a nine year-old. I wanted to get them a playmate. Oreo was starting to suffer from seizures and also had cataracts. He has been my baby from the time he was four months old. I didn't want Georgio to be alone so I thought it was time to introduce a new family member. I thought a Boston Terrier would be a good choice.

I am a volunteer for a no-kill animal shelter and also have been certified to be a Therapy Handler. I have learned so much about dog rescue and have educated myself that I knew this is what I wanted to do.

I read about available dogs on a Boston Terrier rescue site. I finally called and filled out an application. I was visited by one of the volunteers who did a home inspection and filled out a four page document. She turned it in and told me to wait for a phone call from the volunteer who is in charge of placing the rescues.

I remember it was right before the holidays, and I saw two dogs that the rescue site had posted. One was a large brown Boston named Shamus and one was a Boston named Charlie Brown. Charlie Brown was thin in the photo and his story broke my heart. Apparently he was found as a stray in Kern County. He didn't have a chip or any type of identification. In addition, he wasn't fixed.

While he was in the shelter, he acquired kennel cough which can be cured if caught in time with a round of antibiotics. Charlie Brown was adopted while in the shelter but the new owners didn't want to spend the money on curing his kennel cough so they returned him to the shelter. This time the shelter called the Boston Terrier rescue and told them to come and get him or else he would be euthanized. He was picked up and put in isolation where he was treated. He was in bad shape. He could barely stand up and was foaming at the mouth. All I could think was how could they let him get like this? How could the new owners not be willing to spend at least $12.00 and one vet visit to help this animal and how great is this rescue for saving his life? I immediately called the person in charge and told her that I wanted to meet Charlie Brown and Shamus. She told me that I had to bring both of my dogs to meet them as they had to make sure that everyone got along.

I drove from the San Fernando Valley on a Saturday to where the dogs are kept in Orange County which is close to a two hour drive. They were kept at a cage free dog facility where they can run around and play. Once we got there, we met Shamus first and knew right away that Shamus, although sweet and beautiful, might just be too much energy for my IG was going to have surgery on his legs soon. Then we saw Charlie Brown. It was as if he was waiting for us and was looking through the gate. There is a quote that is made by Charlie Brown and he says: "I'll go with you"…I felt as if this is what Charlie was saying to us through his eyes. He was brought to us in the meeting area and immediately he jumped up next to me and started to wag his little stub…I now call it his "mechanical tail". I knew instantly that he was going to be a part of my family. My dogs instantly took to him.

I asked the Boston rescue volunteer to hold him until the following weekend so that I could get everything in order. Normally, when a potential adopter comes to meet a rescue, they go home with the dog. I wanted to be 100% sure that I was making the right decision. Once I left, I couldn't wait until the following weekend to bring him home. Once we got home, he ran into the house and headed right to the Christmas tree…and you guessed it! He christened the branches in the way most male dogs do!!

Charlie continues to bring joy and laughter into my home every day. He easily learned the basic commands and put on all his required weight. The day I decided to rescue Charlie was truly a magical day. I believe that I didn't choose Charlie but that Charlie chose me. I can say that December 25, 2009 was truly a Charlie Brown Christmas.

Learn more about Dina Discola and the animal groups she supports in the "About the Authors" section.

"The dog is the god of frolic."

~ Henry Ward Beecher

I Rescued a Human Today

By Janine Allen

Her eyes met mine as she walked down the corridor peering apprehensively into the kennels. I felt her need instantly and knew I had to help her.

I wagged my tail, not too exuberantly, so she wouldn't be afraid. As she stopped at my kennel I blocked her view from a little accident I had in the back of my cage. I didn't want her to know that I hadn't been walked today. Sometimes the overworked shelter keepers get too busy and I didn't want her to think poorly of them.

As she read my kennel card I hoped that she wouldn't feel sad about my past. I only have the future to look forward to and want to make a difference in someone's life.

She got down on her knees and made little kissy sounds at me. I shoved my shoulder and side of my head up against the bars to comfort her. Gentle fingertips caressed my neck; she was desperate for companionship. A tear fell down her cheek and I raised my paw to assure her that all would be well.

Soon my kennel door opened and her smile was so bright that I instantly jumped into her arms.

I would promise to keep her safe.

I would promise to always be by her side.

I would promise to do everything I could to see that radiant smile and sparkle in her eyes.

I was so fortunate that she came down my corridor. So many more are out there who haven't walked the corridors. So many more to be saved. At least I could save one.

I rescued a human today.

COMPANIONS

"Animals are such agreeable friends
– they ask no questions, they pass no criticisms."
~ George Eliot

Who Chooses Whom?

Some of us have a specific breed or type of cat or dog in mind when we decide that our home needs a new or an additional animal. We may search the internet, shelters and pet stores looking for that special one. Other times, we may not even be consciously thinking about it and a cat wanders in or a dog just shows up. Just who really chooses who?

I believe that somewhere in the universe there must be Angels overseeing a database of animals waiting for that right person who needs the love that only an animal companion can give. When we least expect it, the right one seems to just show up in our life.

Several years ago my friend, Marge had a dog wander into her yard. Her children were all excited about keeping him. Not wanting them to get too attached to a dog that belonged somewhere else, she wouldn't allow them to name him, and so he was referred to as Puppy. Every day the kids could come home from school anxious to see if Puppy was still there. They played with Puppy as they waited to see if someone would come by to claim him. They fought over who got to play with him, feed him and sleep with him. They were always reminded that Puppy may soon be claimed and returned to his rightful home. Thirteen years later, still living with

Marge, Puppy breathed his last breath. He knew from the first day he wandered in that he was in his rightful home.

This story is not over. Puppy was loved generously as each child grew up and eventually left home. The responsibility of taking care of Puppy eventually became Marge's. When Puppy left, she had an empty nest but not for long. Someone else was waiting in the wings to fill the void left by Puppy. Only a day or so after Puppy crossed the rainbow bridge, Harley, a feral cat moved himself right into Marge's home and heart, where he also became part of the family until his final day.

You may have read in other chapters how Tigger and Merlin both came to live in my home. They weren't my first experience of being chosen to be companion to an animal.

When I was a teenager we had several different types of animals on our property. From horses, cattle and various dogs to the wild animals that roamed in the fields and hills around us. Even though our dogs were loving and attentive, I had a long standing fear of getting too close and I wanted something I could snuggle with. I longed for a cat. Nearly every day, I would beg my dad for a cat. I heard the same reply each time, "we don't need a cat, we have enough animals", and my Dad saw no use for a cat to be added to the brood. We had one door that gave the dogs easy access to the outside. Many times it would get accidently closed, so most of my exercise was getting up from the couch to let the dogs in and out. One night, after my usual begging for a cat, we heard a scratch at the front door. Without looking up from his paper, my Dad simply said "go let that animal in and this is the last I want to hear of this cat business." Obediently I went to the door and opened it to let in the dogs that came in one after another and at the end of the parade, followed a beautiful blue-eyed Siamese cat. The dogs didn't seem to notice, or mind, and the cat behaved as if he belonged there. This was quite a surprise; however, I attempted to convince my Dad that it was meant to be. After all, it was at that exact moment I was asking for a cat, and in one walks. Getting to our front door was not a simple task. We had a long driveway up the side of a hill, and the cat had to mingle with all the dogs. Not one to discard any animal, my Dad agreed we could take care of the cat for the night and the next day we would find its rightful home. We posted fliers, placed an ad in our small community newspaper and notified the local vet. We were told that he was a blue-point Siamese cat, and his crossed eyes and kink in his tail were part of his breed. It was difficult to believe that someone wasn't missing him somewhere, but no one showed up to claim him After a few weeks of no results my Dad agreed we could keep him and we named him Si, for Siamese.

Si was a handful at first. Initially we went through gallons of tomato juice to rid him of the skunk odor. The sound of his yowling during the bath, you would think we were skinning him. He brought half-live birds and rodents into the house as gifts, so we weren't allowed to scold him. One day we saw a feral cat wander down our drive way trailed by her kittens, a few which had interesting Siamese markings. It was then my Dad decided that if Si was going to stay, he needed to be neutered.

Si quit romancing the feral cats and skunks after his surgery. He also developed a softer meow which we all appreciated. He ran our property, though, and all the other animals knew it. Si would sit on the arena fence and as the horses would run by during exercise, he would occasionally jump on the back of one and hold on, claws and all. After a while, if he was on the fence, the horses would make a wide berth away from that area. I never saw any confrontation with our dogs. One day, however, a visitor drove up with his dog in the back of his truck. The dog saw Si and leapt from the truck chasing him around the corner of the house. We heard loud whining and ran to find the problem, only to discover the dog penned in a corner up against the house and Si pacing in front of him, tail sharply twitching back and forth and making a very odd guttural sound, never taking his eyes of the dog. I got Si's attention and then removed him from the yard while the dog sulked away and jumped back into the bed of the pickup. A memo must have gone out in the dog world, because that was the last dog to ever chase Si. They all seemed to either avoid him, or at least learned to share the space.

For the remainder of his life, Si kept the barn free of rodents, trained the visiting dogs and kept the horses alert. Even though my Dad had once said he saw no good reason to have a cat, Si won his heart and the two of them could be seen napping together on a lazy afternoon. After Si's passing Dad adopted several cats to take his place. Si had set the bar pretty high. They picked up where Si left off, keeping the barn rodent free and accompanying the dogs when they patrolled the property.

Our lives were changed for the better when Si moved in. He entertained us, kept us company, protected our barn from small intruders and provided us another devoted companion to love.

"If your cat or dog companion thinks

that you are the greatest,

don't seek a second opinion."

Top Reasons to Adopt an Adult Cat

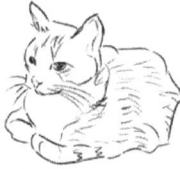

🐾 Adult cats are more mellow. Kittens can be non-stop rambunctious.

🐾 Adult cats don't usually climb your curtains or use your leg as a scratching post.

🐾 Adult cats tend to have a well-developed immune system meaning less visits to the vet.

🐾 Adult cats are very grateful for the second change at a purr-ever home.

🐾 Adult cats are like fine wine, they just get better with age.

🐾 Adult cats are great listeners, and won't repeat your secrets to anyone.

🐾 The **best reason** to adopt an adult cat -
you will save a precious life.

My Wife's Cat

By Bernard J.

My wife, Barbara, and I had been married for over 25 years. We raised a beautiful family together and never let a day go by without saying "I love you". My wife loved cats. Me personally, I couldn't see the value of cats. I couldn't take them on walks, play fetch or other manly things. That aside and being a smart guy, soon after we met, I convinced Barbara I was a great guy when I adopted a cat for her from the local shelter. Molly was definitely my wife's cat. It was a beautiful vision to see my wife curled up in a chair having dozed off from reading a book, and Molly tucked in at her side. Molly was on her lap when we watched TV; watched us from her feeding perch while we ate dinner; and slept near my wife's feet during the night. My wife spared no expense taking care of Molly. If it made my wife happy, it was all right with me. I have never been a cat guy, but sometimes I wondered if my wife had to make a choice between me or Molly, how would I fare?

When my lovely wife was diagnosed with cancer, I did my part to be supportive and do what I could for her; and she went through all the treatments. Every day I would stay by her side, giving her anything she asked for or needed. Next to her at all times, was Molly. Barbara always had one hand near Molly and she seemed so peaceful when Molly would purr.

On a sunny summer day, cancer won and I lost one of the most special parts of my life, and half of my soul. I have never felt so much grief in my life. Family and friends rallied around me for days after her death making sure I had food. When they could find her, they fed Molly and cleaned up after her. Molly was either MIA in the house or she was on top of my wife's side of the bed. I knew at some point I would have to do something about finding Molly another home, but this was all I could do for now. After the crowd of people dwindled to only visiting occasionally, it was my turn to take care of Molly. It seemed like such an inconvenience in my grieving state. Some days when I really didn't care, I could hear my wife's voice reminding me to feed Molly. And I would. But we would just look at each other. My wife used to croon with Molly all the time, but I had never talked to a cat, and I wasn't starting now. So I fed her in silence. My home was overly silent and sad and Molly was too much of a painful reminder of what I had lost. When I came in the bedroom Molly would look at me and slowly get off the bed and hide somewhere.

I didn't have a connection with Molly, and it never occurred to me that she was grieving too.

One night I was sitting on the couch and overwhelmed in my grief, sobbing for my wife, I felt someone touch my knee just like my wife used to. At first I thought it was the memory of my wife reaching out in some odd way through death to comfort me. I opened my eyes and could barely see through the tears. It was Molly sitting next to me and she had placed her paw on my knee. When I looked at her, I felt her sadness too. Nothing could stop the tears. I held Molly and cried into her fur for the longest time. Something changed in me and I saw Molly differently. Our relationship changed and although we aren't the close friends she and Barbara were, she and I are kinda buddies.

I recently sold my home and bought a RV. Molly and I travel around the country doing whatever the day brings. She likes to sit in the passenger seat as I drive, and I talk to her all the time. She doesn't answer back, but then again Barbara didn't much either when I was rambling on while I was driving. And that's all right with me.

Contributed by Bernard J. In Memory of Barbara

Top Reasons to Adopt a Black Dog

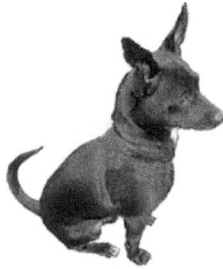

🐾 Black goes with everything. They are easy to accessorize with their harness, collar and leash.

🐾 Black dogs absorb heat... perfect for cozying up to on a cold winter night.

🐾 You get more. Black is a combination of every color in the spectrum, so you will actually have a dog who is blue, green, red, etc.,

🐾 A black dog is just as loving, loyal and trust worthy as any other color.

🐾 Black is slimming. Walking with your black dog, you will appear slimmer. (and enough walking you will become slimmer as well.)

🐾 Black is sexy. Think about it ... black dress, black lingerie....

🐾 Black is unique and valuable ... black pearls, black diamonds.....

🐾 Black is prestigious ... black tie events, black belt martial arts...

🐾 **The best reason -**
Black dogs take the longest
to find a furrever home.
You will save a life, and enhance your own.

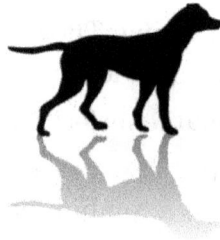

Lancelot

"Look into the eyes of a devoted animal companion
and you will the unbounded GRATITUDE that they feel
for the opportunity they have
to unconditionally love you."[1]

~ Sumner M. Davenport

My devoted companion, Lancelot was pure love. This beautiful white cat was my knight in shining fur, with one blue eye and one gold. He devoted himself to me and my life for 13 wonderful years. He listened to all my stories and kept my secrets. From his cozy spot on the couch by the door, he always greeted me with either a meow or a yawn. We seldom missed a night sleeping together, up until his final day.

His special place to sleep, when not next to me, was under

---

1. excerpt from the book, the "G" spot, the ecstasy of life through GRATITUDE

the covers of the bed. He was the first cat I have ever seen that could tilt the edge of the comforter with his head, and in one smooth move - be on top of the bed, under the covers. I could see the lump that was him cozily curled up, and the remainder of the bed was still smooth and unmoved. The covers would rise and fall softly with each breath in his sleep. After my divorce, he slept on the pillow next to me. His soft snoring kept me company and soothed my then bruised heart. He defied the myth that cat's don't know their name because anytime he wasn't in my lap I could call his name, and he would come right away. He could take an expert leap from the floor and with gliding precision, always land on my full bladder. His favorite game I called fishing for cats. It was a cord attached to a stick with feathers at the end of the cord. Wherever he was in the house, he would know when I picked that up and come running. I could fish him out from under furniture or the closet with that toy. Whether I ran it across the floor or in the air, he played nonstop until he wore me out.

Each night before we went to sleep he would lay on my chest and allow me to scratch him. While he purred we would talk about the day. Actually I did all the talking, he was an excellent listener. He traveled with me everywhere and adjusted to every move I made in my life. Together we languished in the sun of beautiful Cayman Islands, endured traffic jams in Los Angeles, and dodged bullets in Palmdale. He met the animal companions of some of my friends when I would watch their homes when they traveled. He grew to love two dogs, a big golden named Mattie and Lefluer, a little Shih Tzu mix who preferred to be scruffy rather than fluffy. He wasn't fond of their cold noses, but it didn't get in his way when he investigated their food bowl and dinnertime. He would find their tennis balls around the house, grab them with his two front paws and tear into them with his back paws. It always made me laugh. He was such a gentle cat; this was his only resemblance of violent behavior.

At another friend's house, he followed two beautiful Siamese cats, Sydney and Ashley, around the house until they would turn and hiss at him. Then he would position his watch post at the top of the stairs and watch their every move. When Ashley died, he then shared his exclusive window perch with Sydney, until Sydney's final days. Lance was always curious about other cats, but not necessarily enough to want them to join his family. After all, I was his person and he wasn't willing to share my lap.

I am grateful for every time he greeted me as I came in the door, or lifted his head from sleep and yawned at me when I entered the room. I am grateful for every time he jumped on my desk and walked across my keyboard, reminding me that life isn't all about work, and naps are necessary. He taught me that life is in the moments and staring out the window at anything is worth it.

He left me way too soon, after being diagnosed with a 5cm mass in his abdomen which was compromising his pancreas and causing serious problems with his liver and kidney. I used every ounce of my homeopathic knowledge, and every drug the vet thought would help, but his body continued to resist my efforts. He gave up eating on his own three weeks before he passed over. I begged him to eat and fed him with a syringe. I wanted him to live. Because his body was so weak, surgically implanting a feeding tube was not an option. It was too risky. On his final day, he clenched his jaw so tight, it made it impossible for me to feed him with even the smallest syringe. When he not only refused to let me feed him but vomited everything that he put in his mouth, I had to accept it was time and took him to the veterinarian. I kissed him the entire walk from my car to the veterinarian's office, telling him this was his walk of life. He was going to get his healthy life back. He could again play fishing for cats game or kill the tennis balls once played with by dogs. He leaned against me and I felt his purr. He never took his eyes off me during that walk. When I handed him to the Vet, he meowed something at her. My heart hopes he was saying "help me pass over." As he lay in his blanket, ready for what was next, he looked lovingly at Mary and Whitney, his two other human temporary guardians and loving friends. He looked at me again, closed his eyes and then he was gone.

I was devastated at his passing, and I still miss him deeply every day. Even with a new cat now in my home, I still expect to see Lancelot nestled on his blanket on the couch. This is a comfort blanket for me. It held his fragrance for a long time afterwards. I still listen as I work for his cute snoring from the corner of my desk. I was angry for a long time that he was gone. I felt guilty that there had to be something more I could do, or what was it that I didn't do right or enough of? This precious being was my family and more devoted to me than the human family I was born into. He chose his friends wisely and did his best to warn me about certain people. He touched the life of anyone who met him.

I sent him on a journey to a land free from pain, not because I did not love him, but because I loved him too much to force

70

him to suffer by staying here. He still owns real estate in my heart that will remain exclusively his. My life was enriched beyond measure by his love and the lessons he taught me. He paved the journey that led to my better understanding about our animal companions, which led to this book. He was my Knight in shining white fur.

"I believe cats to be spirits come to earth.

A cat, I am sure, could walk on a cloud

without coming through."

~ Jules Verne

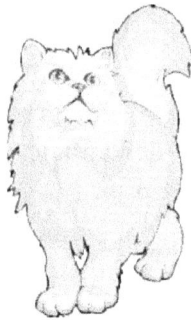

Cats & Children

By Sally Shields

I adore my two cats, who are now nine years old. We met them when they were only two weeks old. The family from whom we were adopting them not only had a big dog that was clomping around the apartment, but a big turtle that went "glub, glub, glub" freewheeling all around the floor, terrorizing the poor dears, I'm sure! When we were finally allowed to take them home at approximately eight weeks, I did everything in my power to reduce the stress of their former life by putting on soft music, petting them slowly and lovingly, having them sleep on the bed with me, and making sure that when they ate, there was a lot of sunlight and fresh water, and no distractions such as the radio or loud music.

Today, we have two human children as well. I fear that my little ones have inadvertently brought back memories of those terrifying large beasts that they had to deal with as infants! I try to eliminate as much aggressive enthusiasm as possible by teaching my children to approach our furry ones slowly and to always leave them alone when they are eating.

My cats are an absolute blessing to me when it comes to reducing my own stress each day! Lafaro is literally my 'mini-me.' She follows me around the house and is almost always within arms-length. If I'm on the couch or at the computer, she's on my lap or the chair next to me. And when I go to sleep, she is my head kitty and Evans is my foot kitty. Head-kitty starts off sharing my pillow, but in the morning I often wake up with her ON my head. My foot kitty is often sleeps at the other end of the bed. It brings down my metabolism to give them love each morning and throughout the day. When I look into my kitties eyes, I see pools of forever. I even had a pet psychic tell me that Lafaro was so connected to me because she was my mother-in-law in a former life. "Who do you think wrote your book for you?" my kitty quipped during a reading. LOL!!!

See "About the Authors" section to learn more about Sally Shields.

"A kitten is in the animal world

what a rosebud is in the garden."

~Robert Southey

My House

By Ellen Bishop

I live in a menagerie, three dogs, a cat, a mouse.
Rhettung chases Landon all about the house.
Apachi nuzzles close to me, sleep closing in.
Zeus snores at Daddy's feet, dawn ready to begin.
Soccer buries his body, quiet in his bed.
Tiny little shavings, covering his head.
Our son sleeps soundly, waiting the new day
It's off to school he'll go, and with friends will play.
Our daughter is now married, a child of her own
Whose tiny sound of laughter brings joy into our home.
Her smile can light a room, for now she cannot crawl.
Long before we know it, she'll leave hand prints on the wall.
I live in a menagerie, three dogs, a cat, a mouse.
Four children always underfoot, yet it's quiet in our house.

See "About the Authors" section to learn more about Ellen Bishop

HEALTH BENEFITS

"Until one has loved an animal,
a part of one's soul remains unawakened."
~ Anatole France

Health Benefits for People with Animal Companions

Every day we learn more about the many health benefits of having animal companions. One study reported at the American Heart Association Scientific Sessions, showed that pets may play a role in taming our physical responses to stress.

After spending only a few minutes with a dog before an upcoming surgical operation, patients have experienced a 37% reduction in their anxiety levels.[4]

Tigger and I walk in the park every day and we have met many people willing to share how their cats and dogs have helped them to improve their health.

Nag, nag nag......we constantly hear that we must exercise for our health. Exercise itself seems boring to some, so having another reason to exercise makes it easier to make the time. People like Steve and Robert have seen the health benefits of exercise with a dog.

Steve told me that he had suffered from high blood pressure for several years. Despite the warnings from his doctor, he just couldn't seem to stay on the diet and exercise program that was prescribed for him. He passes a large park every day on his way to and from home, and he although he had seen several people being walked by their dogs, he kept his old habit of simply sending his dog to the back yard alone to "do his business".

One day a friend told him that this park was a great place to meet women, and dogs are great "chick magnets." That got his attention. So he started taking Bruiser, an overweight Beagle to the park twice a week for a walk. It wasn't long before he discovered his friend was right and there were some "mighty fine looking women" walking dogs in the park. He met friendly people and Bruiser was excited to see the other dogs, so he started walking every day; and then twice a day at the park.

Now he has friends that he meets at the park on a regular basis and the dogs get the chance to socialize as well. It wasn't long before he noticed his clothes were getting a little looser and Bruiser was looking a little more buff too. His next visit to the doctor he was told that his blood pressure was now in the desired range. Within a few months he had also dropped 50 pounds, credited mostly to walking Bruiser every day.

Like many people, Robert runs his small business from home, and is known to spend countless hours on end at his computer without a break. When he agreed to housesit with a friends' dog for a few days, he was suddenly forced to change his schedule to accommodate the dog's need for a walk every few hours.

It was during these breaks from his computer, that Robert discovered this breath of fresh air was what he needed to clear his mind. He found himself more productive in less time when he returned to his work. After his dog-sitting stint was over, he soon felt the loss of this health break. He wasted no time in filling that position with a dog from the local shelter.

At the University of San Francisco they are trying to help alleviate the stresses some students face during final exams, by letting them take a break and spend time with a dog. Law Students can spend 10 minutes petting, playing or just sitting with a dog to help them relieve the stress. According to the school nurse, the animals give off a sense of relaxation, and this exercise has been proven over and again to significantly reduce stress.[5]

The International Journal of Workplace Health Management recently published a study that measured the stress of workers with a dog with them during the work day, against a second group with the same jobs, but without dog companions. Their study revealed that over the course of the day, stress declined for the study group that had their dogs present and increased for the groups without dogs. By the end of the day, a significant difference was found in the stress patterns for the group on the days their dogs were present versus when their dogs were absent. On dog absent days, the person's stress increased throughout the day, mirroring the pattern of the group that did not have a dog.[6]

Some mental health therapists use dogs in therapy. Some people (those not afraid of dogs) appear to feel more at ease with a dog in the room. People often react to the dog in a way that helps the therapist see certain behavior patterns.

Animal companions in the home have been associated with a number of positive health outcomes, including increased survival rates one-year after a heart attack; fewer doctor visits, less loneliness and greater social support. Rescuing a dog from a local shelter could be saving two lives - theirs and yours.

Although some people experience allergies to pet dander, researchers are finding that, a growing number of studies have suggested that kids growing up in a home with "furred animals" -- whether it's a cat or dog companion-- will have less risk of developing allergies and asthma. According to researcher James E. Gern, MD, a pediatrician at the University of Wisconsin-Madison," children in the study had higher levels of some immune system chemicals -- a sign of stronger immune system activation." [7]

"Studies have shown that Alzheimer's patients have fewer anxious outbursts if there is an animal in the home," says Lynette Hart, PhD, associate professor at the University of California at Davis School of Veterinary Medicine.[8]

Walking a dog or just caring for a pet -- for elderly people who are able -- can provide exercise and companionship. On the other hand, cats are ideal pets for seniors who are less mobile, as they are relatively low-maintenance.

According to a Blaire Justice, PhD, a psychology professor at the University of Texas School of Public Health, "Like any enjoyable activity, playing with a dog can elevate levels of serotonin and dopamine -- nerve transmitters that are known to have pleasurable and calming properties."[9]

A study from the University of Minnesota found that those without cats were between 30 and 40 percent more likely to die of cardiovascular disease than those with cat companions. According to lead researcher and neurology professor Adnan Qureshi "The most logical explanation may be that cat ownership may relieve stress and anxiety and subsequently reduce the risk of cardiovascular diseases."[10]

Being with a cat may not actually "cure" depression; however, they may help you get through rough times. When I was going through a very painful and difficult time in my life, I told my cat Lancelot everything. I hugged him and cried into his fur. He stayed relaxed in my arms and simply purred. Even through my tears I could hear and feel his purr. It just seemed to calm me and help me to feel better. As far as I know, he never told my secrets to anyone so he was a safer outlet than the two most popular outlets -- the neighborhood bartender or local hairdresser. Every time he snuggled next to me with loud purrs or snored softly on the pillow next to me in bed, I felt less alone. Some days, I could not help but laugh as he would get himself into one of those contortions that only a cat can do. Laughter is the best medicine against depression. This may not necessarily make logical sense to someone without a cat companion; however, it worked for me. I have heard from others who share their homes with cats, that a cat in the home helps them in staying cheerful as well. It appears that people with cats make fewer visits to health care professionals. Research shows that being able to care for a pet encourages us to take care of ourselves, says Rebecca Johnson, director of the University of Missouri's Research Center for Human-Animal Interaction. [11]

So, if you want to be purrfectly healthy and live a little bit longer, consider sharing your home with an animal companion.

"I love cats because I love my home and after a while they become its visible soul."

~ Jean Cousteau

Top Reasons to Adopt an Older Dog

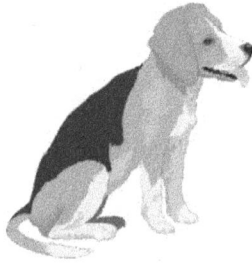

🐾 Older dogs adapt more easily to their new home. Been there - done that.

🐾 Older dogs are house trained.

🐾 Older dogs can be great dude or chick magnets.

🐾 Older dogs have outgrown their destructive puppy behaviors (i.e: chewing on your favorite shoes.

🐾 Older dogs usually know their boundaries and understand what "no" means.

🐾 Older dogs are grateful for the second chance they've been given.

🐾 Older dogs have grown into their full size. What you see is what you get.

🐾 Older dogs don't usually make the same demands on your time as a puppy will.

🐾 You can tell and older dog all your secrets and they won't repeat them.

🐾 The **best reason** to adopt an older dog -
you will save a life.

"A dog reflects the family life.
Whoever saw a frisky dog in a gloomy family,
or a sad dog in a happy one?
Snarling people have snarling dogs,
dangerous people have dangerous ones."
~ Arthur Conan Doyle

Health Benefits for Cats and Dogs with Human Guardians

There are health benefits for cats and dogs living in your home as well. Indoor cats have a tendency to live longer because of lesser exposure to fleas, infectious diseases, hazardous chemicals, poisoned trash and predators. Indoor cats can sometimes live three times longer than an outdoor cat. When you cat is in your home every day, you are more likely to notice changes in their personality and appearance which might be an indication of an illness or injury. If they use a litter box you can see changes in their elimination, which could also alert you to a problem. A friend has indoor/outdoor cats that, while they are faster than the coyotes, come inside at dusk for the remainder of the night. Besides losing a few loved ones over the years to the local wildlife, some of her cats have come home with serious injuries from fights with other cats, or from entanglements in fences. Her injured cat is stressed, and she gets stressed over the vet bills.

Some people believe that indoor cats get lazy and it's cruel not to give them the freedom to roam. Indoor cats that get exercise from interactive toys and play time together can keep your cat active. Monitoring your cat's food instead of a constant full bowl can keep your cat at its purrfect weight. Give your cats a space of their own, where they can go when they need to be alone and feel safe. This could be a corner of a room, or the top of a cat perch. Keep their food separate from their litter box area. Cats, like most people, do not like to eat near their bathroom. Keep your cat's litter box clean, scooping at least once a day and disposing of the deposits outside. Cat's urine is high in ammonia and simply leaving it into your wastebasket can pollute your air and irritate your throat and lungs. Consistent exposure to overwhelming amounts of cat urine ammonia can make you ill. Keeping your home fresh is easier with the ease of clumping cat letter, flushable cat litter ad self-cleaning litter boxes.

Give your cat places to roam in your house or safe garage area. Scratching posts and perches at windows can give your cat the stimulation and satisfaction to their curiosity that they need. Before letting your cat roam in your garage make sure you have cleaned up any poisonous chemicals such as antifreeze. There are new products on the market that can blend in or compliment your home decor as well as satisfy your cat's needs. The cost of cat toys and climbing posts seems to be far less than regular vet visits for serious injuries and infections.

If you do choose to let your cat be an outdoor cat, even partially, make sure that it's spayed/neutered to prevent unwelcomed attention and unwanted litters. Collars help to identify your cat and the safety release type of collar is the best selection. Your identification on the collar will make it easier for your cat to be returned to you if picked up by a stranger or animal control. The safety release is essential in case your cat gets it caught ion something while he's jumping around. Losing the collar is better than the cat losing its life. Check your outdoor cat every night for wounds and scratches, especially puncture wounds from other cat's claws or teeth. Pay close attention to their behavior and look for any changes that might indicate illness or worse, poisoning. When in doubt, consult your veterinarian. It's less stressful to be wrong over a little thing, than wait until it becomes more life threatening and costly.

It's a constant debate whether dogs, especially large ones, should be "outdoor only". According to many veterinarians, dogs are social animals that crave attention; they are usually not happy when they are left alone outside. Dogs left alone in the yard for long periods of time often get bored, lonely and frustrated. As a result, they may develop behavior problems such as barking, digging, escaping, and being overly aggressive. This makes them harder to train.

Free roaming dogs and outdoor only dogs are also more prone to illness and injury from traffic, poisoning, cruelty from passerby's, or fights with other animals. Chronic health problems can develop from cold or heat exposure or untended wounds which isn't always seen in their initial stages because of the human-animal detachment.

If dogs aren't adequately socialized when they're young, they're likely to become fearful or aggressive toward people, and possibly other animals. The reports indicate that people with outdoor dogs tend to be less attached to their dog so these dogs are more easily abandoned and given to shelters. Unsocialized outdoor dogs are more likely to be euthanized.

Having a safe yard for your dog to use for his potty and a place to play, with access to indoor space with his people - the ideal life for a dog. However that isn't always possible. Creating a happy medium is important for the health and stress of both animal and person. It starts with selecting the right dog for your home and lifestyle. Regardless of whether a dog is inside or outside, training is essential. Time spent training your dog insures against future problems.

If your dog is going to be primarily outside, make sure his environment is safe, and he knows his boundaries without having to be chained or tied to a post. Make sure to provide a safe, escape-proof shelter, fresh water and shade from summer sun and warmth from winter cold. Provide busy toys and human interaction often.

Some people believe that a keeping their dog outside all the time, is their best protection against intruders. Bill told me that thought this too, until that premise was put to the test. He felt his home was very safe because his Doberman, Hamlet, would bark at anyone who walked by. The closer they were to his fenced, the more vicious his dog behaved. Bill felt that anyone seeing this would think twice about trying to come in his yard.

Bill came home one night to find something he believed would never happen. His house had been burglarized. He found out that it looked like, one person kept the dog distracted and two others climbed the opposite fence and entered his house. One of his neighbors finally became irritated at his dog barking and noticed what looked like someone teasing the dog. They yelled at this man and he ran away, but they didn't think to call the police. During this time, after getting thousands of dollars of his valuables, the intruders were able to escape through his back yard. The fence was partially broken at the spot they used.

Bill later heard from local security company that a lone dog is easy for an intruder to disarm or overcome. Plus, dogs are territorial. If their territory is only the yard, the intruder who is able to get into your home will have the advantage over the dog. After all the dog is not allowed into your home, so the chance of them going after an intruder in your home is slim. Hamlet was always left in the yard.

Unsocialized dogs can be a potential hazard to visiting friends and family, especially children who might be playing in your yard. If you are looking for a guard dog, there are several organizations that can assist you in selecting, training and properly housing your dog.

Cats and dogs thrive and behave better when living indoors with their human family members. Less injury and illness in your animals can equal less stress on you and them emotionally; and less stress on your bank account.

My Running Partner

By Victoria Loveland-Coen

Experts have been telling us for decades now that aerobic exercise is vital to not only our physical health, but our mental health as well. The endorphins released during prolonged exercise have a profound calming effect on our nervous system. Hence, we are more relaxed and better able to handle stressful situations.

Running outdoors...preferably in nature...has always been my choice for aerobic exercise, and I've benefitted from its effect it for years. With the exception of a good pair of shoes, running doesn't require any special equipment or location, and you don't need to schedule a partner or team to do it. Yes, there are days when I have to drag myself out there and, occasionally it's uncomfortable, but when I return home I feel so darn good, it was worth the effort. Any remaining stress just pours out with the sweat and after a shower I'm relaxed, rejuvenated and ready for anything.

About 15 years ago a new dimension of enjoyment entered my running experience. For the first time in my adult life, we got a puppy. My husband and I named her Willow. Willow was an energetic, rambunctious puppy (oh, aren't they all at that age?) and she needed daily exercise. What a perfect opportunity for us both! She needed to be run and I needed to run. What a joy! When we returned, she would settle down and sleep for a good part of the day so I could work.

I've heard it said that exercise is the thing dogs crave most...even more than food. It makes sense. They're built to run. Unfortunately, many dogs are left in their apartments or houses for far too long and don't get the opportunity to release their energy. This has got to cause tension and stress to build up in their little bodies. No wonder they often get into mischief, and become destructive in the house when their owners are away! It's kind of how my children are when they don't get enough exercise. They get antsy, jittery, stressed and can often be destructive.

Running with an animal on a leash took some getting used to, but after a time (and after she grew a little older) we developed this amazing rhythm. Our strides began to match and we moved together in beautiful symmetry. Horseback riders often describe the unity they feel when riding...the horse and rider become one unit. That's exactly how I feel running with my dog...with the added benefit of my getting exercise along with my pet.

I lost sweet Willow two years ago, and there was a deep void in my life for many months. Running was not the same for me without her. I kept looking for her beside me and seeing nothing. I stopped running altogether for a time.
Fortunately someone told me about a rescue dog that needed

a good home, and after five minutes visiting with this dog, our whole family fell in love. She's a German Shepherd/Golden Retriever mix. A big dog. And I'm happy to report that Aurora has taken over where Willow left off.

Aurora is now my running buddy. We developed a synchronistic rhythm rather quickly. When I feel a boost of energy and want to run a little faster, she immediately picks up the pace. When I'm pooping out and want to slow down and walk for a bit, without missing a stride, she's right there with me. Several times during our run she, of course, needs to stop do her business, or just sniff. In the beginning, this would irritate me, as it forced me to stop. But now, I view these moments as an opportunity to rest and take in the beauty around me. I'll often notice how the sun hits a few leaves in a certain way as they glisten with an impossibly vibrant green. Or I'll hear birds, and then have the chance of looking up and observing them soar overhead. I suddenly feel so grateful for the opportunity of being there in that moment, for my dog, and for the magnificent beauty of this amazing planet.

You must give this a try with your dog to really see what I mean. For the best experience try running in nature. It will enhance the stress-reducing experience at least ten-fold. Is there a forest or a beach close to where you live? Is there a mountain trail, or a shady bike path? If getting out into nature is not convenient, find a park and run there. You will find the combination of being surrounded by natural beauty, running in rhythm with your dog, and allowing the endorphins to course through your body the most joyous, peaceful, relaxing and invigorating experience you'll ever feel.

And that feeling will continue to spread waves of peace throughout your day... and your dog's as well.

See "About the Authors" section to learn more about Victoria Loveland-Coen.

"The greatest pleasure of a dog is that you may
make a fool of yourself with him
and not only will he not scold you,
but he will make a fool of himself, too."
~ Samuel Butler

If I Knew Then What I Know Now

By Marcia Klark.

You know how we always says, if I only knew then what I know now..., we would do things differently? I say that today.

A few years ago I left a very abusive relationship. I hid the abuse from everyone. It seemed that no one noticed that I was jumpy all the time and more short tempered. I worked hard to please everyone, even in my relationship, but it seemed like I couldn't do anything right. I wasn't sleeping well, and I was tired all the time. I would cry at the drop of a hat.

Then one night I couldn't pee, even though it felt like I really had to. I had had bladder infections when I was younger, but this felt much worse, I was in real pain. I had to drive myself to the emergency room, where they diagnosed me with a kidney infection, most likely brought on by stress and lack of proper hydration. As soon as they gave me medicine and fluids, I felt better physically. When the doctor started to ask me questions, I couldn't stop crying and I know I wasn't making any sense. He recommended I stay the night for observation and they gave me something to help me sleep. When I woke up 12 hours later, I felt better than I had in months and I seem to have a clearer head. A psychiatrist visited me that morning and suggested I needed to make some changes in my life, and he gave me the phone number of a therapist, who later put me on antidepressants.

When I went home, I not only didn't get any compassion for my infection, I was yelled at for the money the hospital visit was going to cost even though we had insurance. A few days later, I moved out. Since I hadn't told anyone of my ordeals in this relationship, my family wasn't supportive of the split and friends turned their back on me. What I thought would be a good new beginning for me was instead very lonely. Without any help, I found a new home and a second job. For a few days, I felt scared but empowered, then the fear kicked in. Did I do the right thing? Was I over exaggerating the situation like everyone was saying? I couldn't afford to see the therapist and pay for my Prozac too, so I opted to just buy the drugs and deal with the depression by myself. I could get myself to work. I used to love my job but now I didn't seem to enjoy it anymore. I faked it on the outside so everyone would think I was ok. After work I would go home and have a few drinks and go to bed. I know now that alcohol is an depressant, and shouldn't be taken with Prozac, but I was just trying to get through the night. A couple of friends would call, but I could hear that they were tired of my misery and after telling me to quit feeling sorry for myself and stop the pity party, they didn't stay on the phone long. I didn't know how to get out of my funk, and I felt very alone.

Then one Saturday I took my usual trip to the grocery store. In front of the store was a group of people with animals from a local rescue group. They were having an adoption day. One beautiful cat really caught my eye, and I stopped to coo at her. One of the volunteers asked if I wanted to adopt her but I'd never had a pet and my apartment building didn't allow pets, so I said "No" even though I was really drawn to the cats. So the volunteer suggested maybe I could be a volunteer so I could be around the cats when I had time. For some reason it clicked with me and I signed her form. Later after I got home, I started to regret saying yes to the idea. The first time the group person called me I didn't return her call. The second time she called I was napping and answered the phone without thinking. She was so cheerful, even when I said I wasn't sure if I could do it. She nicely persuaded me to just come to an orientation and see what I thought. It took all the strength I had to go to the meeting but I did.

Something that meeting felt right so I signed up as a cat volunteer. All I had to do was sit with them, play with them and clean up their areas if I wanted to. I was there for the rest of that day and the entire next day. Just being with the cats made me feel better. They all seemed to love me just for being there. I didn't have to do anything to try to please them; in fact, they helped me pet then by walking under my hand or rubbing up against me. And all that purring was pure music to my heart. For weeks I would go to the shelter and sit with the cats. It may sound funny, but I'd take a book and read aloud to them. They just sat around me and seemed to be a great audience. They needed me to be there to show them love and I needed the love they so freely gave.

It was a few weeks when I had a sudden realization. I hadn't had a drink since my second visit with the cats. I was feeling lighter and happier for no specific reason at all. Work was fun again. I didn't seem to be faking being happy as much. I kept going back to the cats. Just because I couldn't have a cat at home didn't mean I couldn't have cats in my life.

I bought my last prescription for Prozac six months later and with the help of a new therapist, slowly detoxed myself from it, and I haven't had the need to go back. My therapist helped me to really learn about my life and see more good things about myself and she has helped me to understand how helping the cats is really helping myself.

Some of the cats that come to the shelter have been abused and neglected by the people they trusted. It was another ah-ha moment for me. Taking care of these cats help me to realize that just because someone didn't love them and take proper care of them, didn't mean they weren't worthy of love. It is the abuser who has the problem, not the victim. These cats couldn't stand up for themselves against the abuse and I was afraid to stand up for myself. I was learning about myself by loving these sweet furry friends. I had never thought that being a volunteer could be so meaningful and make such a difference in both sides of the equation.

Today I make different choices in my relationships and even how I talk with my family. Even if they don't believe me, I still tell them the truth about what happened then and what I am doing now.

If I knew then what I know now, the only things I would do differently, would be to get out of the bad relationship at the first sign of danger, tell people the truth about what was going on, and get involved with cats sooner.

"Time spent with cats is never wasted."

~ Sigmund Freud

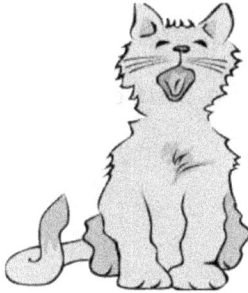

Handle Stress Like a Cat

If it moves, play with it
If it appears to be in the way -
know that is only an illusion.
If it bothers you, walk away.
When in doubt - sleep on it
Sing your own song.

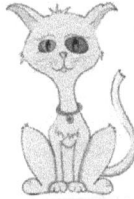

Handle Stress Like a Dog

If you can't eat it or play with it.

Pee on it and walk away.

Wag your tail

and the rest of the body will join in the fun.

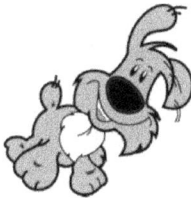

If a Dog Were Your Teacher

You would learn things like:

🐾 When loved ones come home, always run to greet them.

🐾 Never pass up the opportunity to go for a joyride.

🐾 Allow the experience of fresh air and the wind in your face to be pure ecstasy.

🐾 Take naps.

🐾 It's okay to drool in your sleep.

🐾 Stretch before rising.

🐾 Run, romp, and play daily.

🐾 Thrive on attention and let people show their affection

🐾 Avoid biting when a simple growl will do.

🐾 On warm days, stop to lie on your back on the grass.

🐾 On hot days, drink lots of water and lie under a shady tree.

🐾 When you're happy, dance around and wag your entire body.

🐾 Delight in the simple joy of a long walk.

🐾 Be loyal.

🐾 Never pretend to be something you're not.

🐾 If what you want lies buried, dig until you find it.

🐾 When someone is having a bad day, be silent, sit close by, and nuzzle them gently.

🐾 ENJOY EVERY MOMENT OF EVERY DAY!

Another advantage of big picture windows in a home: the dogs and cats don't have to move so often to stay sleeping in the patch of sunlight on the floor."

~ Original Author Unauthenticated

"Animals are such agreeable friends -
they ask no questions;
they pass no criticisms."
~ George Eliot

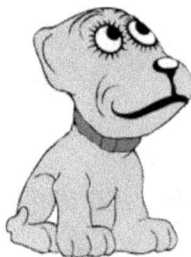

LOVING CARE

"A cat has absolute emotional honesty:
human beings, for one reason or another,
may hide their feelings,
but a cat does not."
~ Ernest Hemingway

Spay and Neuter

In the US we end the lives of hundreds of thousands of little angels in fur every week. These animals lose their lives on the highways, in unprotected yards and the local pound. Between 3 and 4 million adoptable animals are euthanized in animal shelters each year simply because they do not have homes. ***These animals did nothing wrong, other than to be born.*** Someone then lost interest in them; didn't want the responsibility for them anymore; couldn't (or wouldn't) afford to take care of them anymore; a choice was made between a new boy/girl-friend and the animal; a decision was made to move to a new home that didn't allow animals and many more reasons.

Yet, hundreds of dogs and cats have litters every day because they are not spayed or neutered. The discussion on this topic can sometimes be heated. At a recent business gathering one man said he would never cut the balls off his dog because he didn't want a sissy dog. Some studies show that intact dogs do have a tendency to be more aggressive, however, it's an urban legend that sterilized dogs become docile, fat and lazy. Professional dogs, such as police dogs are intact, however, they are trained to use their aggression responsibly. An aggressive, untrained dog can be a costly hazard. Walking my dog this morning, two people walking unneutered dogs approached each other, and the two dogs immediately lunged at each other and a fight began. After the people succeeded in untangling the dogs, both the people and the dogs had injuries. Both people exasperatedly claimed that "their dog was friendly" and "don't know how this happened."

Another woman said just because she wasn't going to have children, she wasn't going to remove her ovaries and she feels the same about her cat. When her cat goes into heat she locks the cat in a closet, adding that it's a large walk-in closet. So I nicely asked if someone locked her in a closet when she had her time of the month. My question wasn't appreciated, although a few people around me snickered. Even the most protected house cat can accidently escape and find a temporary breeding partner.

When volunteering at a local shelter, I met a small dog that had developed mammary tumors because she had not been spayed. Her owners dumped her at the shelter because they didn't want to deal with a dog with tumors, even though they admitted that their Vet had warned them of this possibility with this breed, if they didn't get her spayed. Fortunately, this shelter made a commitment to this dog to pay for the surgery to fix her tumors and also to get her spayed. Then they found her a new loving, furrever home.

When I was a child we had a collection of animals. My Dad, being a good cowboy made sure all our dogs, horses and working stock were sterilized before bringing them home. Even when a stray cat came to live with us, as soon as time passed when no one came to claim him, he was neutered. That made a dent in the population explosion he had been causing with the feral cats living in the nearby mountains. I've read several arguments on the health issues of spaying/neutering. Some say additional health problems occur when an animal is not sterilized and others cite stories of health problems when they are. Some animal health care experts are citing a new study that shows that neutering early may lead to health issues in giant breed dogs later in life.[12] Unfortunately, some people may use this as their excuse to not sterilize their dog at any time.

News stories continue to report that more animals suffer the risk of death because of the over population of cats and dogs. Our kill rate at shelters is on the rise. People are still abandoning their animals at the side of the road and some drive them to the shelters (I was told that owner relinquished animals are the first in line to be euthanized at the pound.) People still allow their dogs and cats to roam neighborhoods freely to act at the whim of nature and the homeless pet population continues to rise.

The real heart of the issue is the irresponsible people.

A man in my neighborhood was going to breed his little dog so each of his children would have a pet of their own. That idea changed when he calculated how much it would cost to take care of that many more dogs. It was cheaper to spay his dog so his pocketbook made the decision. I heard another story where a woman wanted to have her cats bear a litter so her children could witness the miracle of birth. This spurred an angry response from the person she was talking with, that she should then also take her children to the local pound so they could experience the miracle of needless death.

Many people cite financial reasons for not spaying/neutering, even though there are locations in nearly every city that have low cost and sometimes free spay/neuter clinics. Some areas will fix certain breeds of dogs at any time for no charge. Many areas offer discount on the rabies shots and exams when an animals is sterilized..

If money is the issue, two online resources maintain databases of low cost and sometimes free spay and neuter clinics. They are listed in the Resources section of this book.[13]

My decisions today are still influenced by the care and decisions my Dad displayed towards the animals he chose to bring home. It is now also strongly influenced by the number of dead animals I see by the side of the road hit by a car. Add to that, the stories I hear from people who work at kill shelters and no kill rescues.

These angels in fur enter our lives and look to us as their guardians; to make the decisions that will contribute to making their lives happier, healthier and filled with love. In return they love us unconditionally. If you were your dog or cat, what would you want?

Cute video on YouTube: Take me to the Clinic:
http://www.youtube.com/watch?v=CMzW3LIkNLA

Doing the Right Thing

Los Angeles County, as many other areas, has a mandatory Spay/Neuter law. The purpose of this law is to attempt to control the over population of stray dogs and cats. The rescues and shelters are overcrowded and the number of innocent cats and dogs being euthanized continues to rise.

When he was old enough, my veterinarian recommended that Merlin visit one of the mobile spay/neuter clinics. One was conveniently scheduled regularly at a nearby neighborhood. A call the day before resulted me an appointment for Merlin, which meant I had to walk Tigger earlier than usual to make the scheduled time. Tigger loved the early morning air, and Merlin had no clue how this day was going to change the rest of his life.

When I arrived, there was a small crowd lined up all for the same time. The clinic took in all the animals first thing in the morning and then performed the surgeries one after the other. We were to be called when our pet was ready to be picked up in the afternoon.

This particular mobile clinic offered both free and fee services. If a person could show their income was below a certain amount, they could receive the services for free, otherwise it was $100. As I waited my turn in line, a woman ahead of me was explaining that she had rescued her two cats from an area near her home and she didn't have the heart to take them to the pound because she was afraid they would be euthanized. She had tried a local no-kill shelter, but they wanted an intake fee which she couldn't afford. Her daughter convinced her that these cats had chosen their family, so they must keep them. They had all quickly become very attached to these furry little angels so she was at the clinic to have them sterilized.

The intake technician informed her that her income was a little over the annual income limit for free services and she would have to pay the $100 fee per cat. She kept attempting to explain that she didn't have that much money. Even though her income appeared to be above what they considered the "low income" level, she was struggling to pay her bills. She wanted to do the right thing for these cats.

No amount of tears or begging would change the technician's mind. He was following the rules and he couldn't budge. Fortunately, someone in line, hearing this story stepped up and paid the fee for her two cat's surgery. Some might argue that if she couldn't pay the surgical fee she shouldn't have the cats; whereas others would say she was showing great love for these animals by taking them in and attempting to do what was in their best interests. Regardless of outside opinions, this woman was following her heart and doing what she felt strongly was the right decision for her life and her family.

The mandatory spay/neuter law has become controversial. One reason is the cost. Many people are struggling to meet their financial obligations. Being forced to make a choice between paying their utilities or groceries or use that $100 to sterilize their animal feels like a losing proposition either way. County veterinarians are supposed to report any animal that is brought in intact unless provided proof that the animal meets one of the exemptions. It is believed that many intact pets fail to get the veterinary care they may need because people fear the consequences. Granted, there are those that will ignore any law or refuse to get their pet sterilized for a variety of reasons; however, for those that are showing up to do the right thing and are struggling financially, there must be some leeway. The inflexibility this woman was facing could have resulted with these two cats contributing later on to the pet overpopulation.

I'm in support of humanely reducing the number of pets that roam our streets and fill our shelters, living limited life spans without being part of a loving family. Responsible spay/neutering is one way. Taking the time to consider how financially difficult it is for many families at this time; and being humane in the treatment towards those who show up attempting to do the right thing is also important. We must look at the consequences we create, when we draw such a hard line decision and refuse to consider alternatives.

You may know Betty White from her many years on television. Her dedication to animals is no secret. She shares the same concern as many of us about the pet overpopulation problem. Betty has joined with Actors for Animals to raise funds to provide free spay/neuter services to as many animals as possible. Although over population is no joke, she calls this program "Bucks for Balls", asking for a simple $1 donation to make a difference.

You can find out more about this program on the Actors & Others for Animals website listed in the resource section of this book.[14]

"I had been told that the training procedure with cats was difficult. It's not. Mine had me trained in two days."

~ Bill Dana

Only My Dog!

By Katie W.

Last year, I lost a very dear friend of mine. We had been friends from high school. We did so much together. We even went to the shelter to adopt dogs from the same litter, brother and sister. We named them Grant and Gracie. We took our Chihuahuas everywhere and spoiled them with all things little dog.

Grant was Cyndi's dog and he was very devoted and protective of her. He sat next to her or on her lap, slept next to her in bed and followed her wherever she went. He would growl at anyone who tried to pet him, or get too close to her. Even the vet had to tranquilize Grant to exam him when he was sick one time. Cyndi did his grooming and even cut his nails. I wasn't as brave and took Gracie to a local groomer whom she seemed to like.

As a stay at home mom, Grant and Cyndi were together all the time. She seldom left him home when she went out, because he would howl until she returned. She thought his devotion and protective behavior was cute, and I envied her because Gracie was devoted to me, but not nearly as much. My kids could feed Gracie, but she growled if they wanted to pet her too much, and she didn't care much for my husband. She liked her groomer and tolerated our veterinarian. My husband didn't like Gracie in the bed, so her bed was on my night table. This way she could see me and be close.

Cyndi was killed in a car accident and the shock was overwhelming to all of us. While her family and friends dealt with the loss, her daughters took turns trying to take care of Grant. Cyndi had always been the one to feed him, so he was rather vicious when they tried to put the food in his dish. They had to wait until he was out of the room, fill his dish and then wait for him to find it later. Grant went from room to room and howled non-stop for Cyndi. On top of their grief, Grant was grieving too and no one could do anything for him. In a few short days, he became even more aggressive and scared.

No one knew what to do. At first I thought maybe I could take Grant and he would adjust to my home with Gracie. Even though Grant and Gracie were siblings, he wasn't always nice to her. He treated me with the same scary reaction as he did everyone, except Cyndi. Now, he was losing weight and howling almost non-stop. Everyone was grieving the loss of Cyndi and losing more sleep because of Grant. We asked vets and trainers what to do, but every suggestion they gave us failed with Grant. He wanted Cyndi and no one else.

Finally, based on advice from the vet, the family made the sad decision that Grant would have to be put down. It was like losing a final part of Cyndi. They put a mild sedative in a spray bottle and sprayed some in the air. Since he wasn't eating, they couldn't put it in his food. Finally he breathed in enough sedative and when he was asleep, they placed him in the carrier and took him to the vet. Finally he be back with Cyndi - in heaven. Everyone cried.

Watching what Grant went through and the torment on Cyndi's family, it no longer seemed cute that Grant was such an only one-person dog. It started me thinking about what might happen to Gracie if anything happened to me. Would my family be able to take care of her? Would she let them? I couldn't stand the thought of my family going through what Cyndi's family just did, at any time.

I made calls and interviewed several trainers until I found one that trained with positive reinforcement. She worked with us for several months. My entire family, including my, at first reluctant, husband, put in all the time and effort that was required to make this work. We started by me placing Gracie between me and my someone else on the couch, so she was sitting equally between both of us. I would take my daughters hands and let Gracie see me use their hands to pet her. She received ongoing praise and sometimes a special treat every time she relaxed and let herself be petted by someone other than me. We don't use treats all the time because I don't want her to get fat or rely on getting treats every time. It was hard for me, at first to let go and let other people touch and feed Gracie, but my goal of having her be a well-adjusted family dog was always on my mind. My husband and daughters took turns feeding Gracie, and Gracie watched as I stood by and their hands placed the food in her dish. They talked nicely to her when they fed her and while she ate. We took turns walking Gracie together. I would usually start out and part way on the walk, give the leash to whoever was walking with me, telling Gracie she is a good girl all the time.

Gracie bed was moved to the floor so she no longer had an eye level view of me when we sleep. A few times I would move her bed into one of my daughter's rooms during the day, so she could nap in there. I started by sitting in the room, usually reading a book so I was nearby even though we were in a different room.

Now I have a permanent bed for her in each of my daughter's rooms as well as the living room and my bedroom. This way we got her accustomed to being in any room with any member of my family. One of our greatest surprises was one night when we were all in the living room after dinner. My daughter had taken her to the back yard for a quick potty. When they came back in, Gracie jumped on the couch and onto my husband's lap. She curled up and lay down just like it was a normal thing to do. We tried not to get too excited and scare her. She only stayed there a minute, and then she came to my lap.

Little by little, she has welcomed every member of my family into her heart. We use some of these same techniques when my friends come to visit. She has her favorites and doesn't like everyone. I think this is acceptable since not all my friends are as much a dog lover as I am, and maybe Gracie knows that. She's entitled to her opinions. As long as she fits with my family first and foremost, we are happy.

"As anyone who has ever been around a cat
for any length of time well knows,
cats have enormous patience
with the limitations of the human kind."
~ Cleveland Amory

Charlie

By Ellen Bishop

Running across the grassy yard, he skids to a halt
Bouncing around like a pup and throwing his ball
Intelligent and handsome, so well behaved
A brand new home with two children to play
His gentle heart weakened by heartworm disease
Could have been negated for a very small fee
He passed from this world during treatment and care
Leaving our lives with a gaping hole there
For the health of your pets, on preventative start
Remember Charlie and protect their hearts.

Charlie was probably the most personable, docile, beautiful Doberman I have ever seen. He had a show ring build, docked tail and ears, shiny coat and sparkling eyes. He was owner surrendered to the shelter, due to the failing health of the owner. From the moment he walked through our doors, the entire staff was totally in love with him. He would bound across the yard when we let him out to play in the warm spring sun chasing the closest ball we had thrown for him.

Unfortunately, Charlie tested heartworm positive. One of the dangers owners neglect is heartworm preventative due to lack of knowledge or funds for the medications. We knew this would make it more difficult to find him a home but we were determined. We tried Doberman rescues, foster homes, and then finally the decision was made to put him up for adoption at our shelter.

One day about two months later, a family arrived that would end up taking this wonderful guy home with them. They took him out to play with their young children to ensure that he was compatible with everyone in the household. Charlie paid attention to the little ones more than the adults, lying on his belly for them to climb on him, kissing their faces and wiggling in excitement. This continued each day for a week, with the family making certain this was the dog for them. Eventually, they finalized the adoption and took Charlie home with the understanding that he must return for his neuter and heartworm treatments at the end of the week.

Once in his new home, Charlie had a recurrence of kennel cough and his surgery was postponed for a month while his body fought the infection and regained strength. When he returned he was even more loving than previously, greeting each of us with wiggles and kisses. The love he was being shown in his home gleamed in his gorgeous brown eyes.

The following morning, our vet listened to his heart and lungs, hearing nothing to cause alarm and we proceeded with his anesthesia. I prepared him for both the neuter and heartworm treatments, laid him on the surgery table, and began prepping the next animal in line. He sailed through without any apparent complications, then was placed back into his kennel for monitoring and warmed with blankets. We kept a close eye on him for the first three hours, noticing no signs to cause alarm. After finishing all the scheduled surgeries for the day, the suite was cleaned, laundry completed, floors mopped, and we went about our other duties, leaving just two hours before closing for the night.

I set to work heartworm testing more dogs for adoption, checking on the surgery animals after an hour. Charlie was still sleeping soundly, a steady rhythmic breathing pattern, mild eye reflex and a good heart beat. I went to feline leukemia testing the cats that would be available for adoption the next day. Once this chore was finished, I again went back to check on Charlie and settle him in for the night. His next round of heartworm treatment would be tomorrow. I made sure he had his eyes open enough to move around a little, gave him fresh blankets, turned on a small heater, gave him a little food and water, then shut off the lights and locked the door for the night.

Shortly after clocking in the following morning, I did my usual task the day after surgery; checking on any animals left over night for additional treatments. I turned on lights and opened doors as I went, talking with some of the long term residents, greeting new visitors, and scratching a few ears or giving treats along the way to puppies. I was not prepared for what would greet me in the surgery suite. Charlie had passed away during the night, curled in a ball to sleep with his nose resting on his hip. He looked so quiet that we knew his heart simply failed to continue beating.

I reached for my cellular phone, calling Dr. Jennifer at once to notify her of the situation and take her orders for his body. She asked the usual battery of questions, which I checked, then responded to her. We determined later in the day after her arrival that Charlie's heart had simply been too weak from the heartworm overload to continue beating. It was such a terrible shame that a disease that could have been prevented with the proper medicine would take such an outstanding animal from our midst. Thank goodness he died in his sleep peacefully. I don't know how we would have borne the weight if he had struggled with no one there to help him.

Dr. Jennifer contacted Charlie's parents, made them aware of the situation, and asked their wishes with regards to his body. Even after only having him such a short time, they had fallen in love with this boy and made the decision to have him cremated and returned to them. It was a true testament to what a family will do for the right dog who became a member so quickly.

See the Authors section at the back of the book to learn more about Ellen Bishop

Foxtails

As we were doing the final editing of this book, I re-read Charlie's heartworm story. Tigger had now been in my home for a year. Even though I had taken him to the vet several times for his tummy and his routine shots, he had not been tested for heartworm. I heard several opinions from friends regarding whether they test or not. Heartworm is more prevalent in areas of swampy and standing water, and humid places like the East Coast. I decided better to be safe than sorry and with an inexpensive blood test, at least I would know.

The test results were good - no heartworm. While he was there the vet did her basic eyes, ears, teeth exam and noticed he had something in his ear. She questioned if he had been shaking his head or scratching at his ears. I later learned that a foxtail within the ear canal causes head shaking or ongoing scratching.. He scratched one ear, maybe once a week, but nothing regularly and he didn't act like he was trying to get something out of it. After a deeper exam and using a probe she found he had 1/2" fox tail embedded in the wax in his ear. Further exam produced another one from his other ear. He was lucky that his ear wax prevented the fox tails from getting to the ear drum.

Foxtails are grass-like weeds which resemble the tails of foxes and are usually found only in states west of the Mississippi. Once embedded, foxtail seeds cause severe infections and abscesses. I've picked these prickly things off my pants when I hike certain trails. I knew what they looked like but I have not noticed them anywhere around my neighborhood or other places that I have taken Tigger; until one day when I found bushes of them around the parking lot of one of the pet stores Tigger and I visit. It appears the gardeners attempt to keep them trimmed, however, now knowing the bushes are there, I avoid that side of the parking area.

It's a benefit that he has such short hair because longer and thicker haired dogs seem to get more of them embedded in their fur and skin. If I ever see one sticking in his fur, I've been instructed how to carefully pull it straight out, making sure not to break it off in the process.

Sometimes Tigger likes to eat grass. I've been told that foxtails can be ingested this way as well. After this experience, if he appears to have a problem swallowing or trying to clear his throat after eating grass, he'll be to the vet as soon as possible! Stories I read explain that waiting can only make foxtails harder to find, allow it to migrate and become more dangerous and make treatment more difficult.

I hadn't known about the dangers of foxtails. Now that I do, I am more diligent in watching where we walk and where he sticks his head.

If a Cat Were Your Teacher

You would learn things like:

🐾 Stretch before rising.

🐾 Always enjoy the sunbeams.

🐾 Thrive on attention and let people show their affection.

🐾 Find joy in the little things.

🐾 Every loving act deserves a purr-fect compliment.

🐾 Don't stress the small stuff, and jump over the big stuff.

🐾 Be curious, you never know what good is waiting through the next door.

🐾 Never pretend to be something you're not.

🐾 Take Naps.

🐾 Clean your inner and outer self often. (especially before someone else does it for you.)

🐾 When in doubt, look at it from a different perspective.

🐾 There is always time for play.

🐾 Accept that sometimes you can see things that others cannot.

🐾 When someone is having a bad day, be silent, sit close by, and express only love.

🐾 ENJOY EVERY MOMENT OF EVERY DAY!

"Cats seem to go on the principle that it never does any

harm to ask for what you want."

~ Joseph Wood Krutch

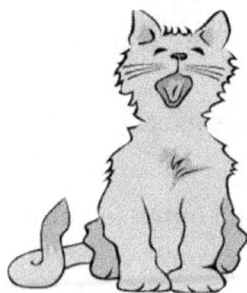

NUTRITION
&
HEALTH

*"Any glimpse into the life of an animal
quickens our own and makes it so much
the larger and better in every way."*
~ John Muir

Television shows, articles and some medical professionals continue to advise us to read the labels and become aware of the nutrients (or lack thereof) in the foods we eat. As people become busier with their work and social life, they look for shortcuts to give themselves more time. One time saver is usually resorting to fast food instead of a quality nutritious meal, for both themselves and their human and animal family.

It's not uncommon to hear someone say, "Cats and dogs can eat anything." It may appear that some have an iron stomach. When they are fed processed food full of by products and chemicals, their digestive system may appear to become tuned to junk food, just like humans, however, researchers report that junk food can make our body retain more fat, invite medical problems and shorten our lives. Just like humans - animals are what they eat.

Some cats and dogs will react more drastically to certain foods and ingredients than others. Each day I meet more people whose cats and dog companions have been diagnosed with a food allergy. No diet is universal.

When I was growing up, our animals (dogs, cats, chickens, horses and cattle) were all fed food that was either raised or grown on our land. Our freezer was filled each year with fresh beef and pork so our dogs ate much of the same fresh, home-grown, protein that we did. It wasn't until years later living on my own in the city, when I adopted my first cat, that I was faced with the decision on what to feed him. Most of my friends fed whatever was the cheapest or most advertised brand available at the grocery. We trusted the stores would only carry what was best for us and our animals.

For the past several years we have become more educated on the importance of what we eat. It is equally as important to read the labels on the foods we feed our animal companions. Being conscious about the foods we all eat - human and animal - can help us to see how food affects our health and stress.

On her radio show, Dr. Kim talks weekly about how and why nutrition is a huge factor in the health of our animals. It's this way for humans, so why would we think it's any different for our cats and dog companions. Stress can affect the immune system and cause a propensity for disease; and being ill can cause more stress.

When I first brought Tigger home as a foster, he came with a supply of the food they had been feeding him at the shelter. I obediently fed him this same food during his time as a foster dog in my home. It was important that I maintained the same diet he had been on at the shelter. Doing this, he would then go to his furrever home with his stomach already tuned a diet that would be easy for his furrever guardians to maintain.

At first everything seemed great, and then every few weeks I was alerted to the sound of him vomiting. When I would take him for a walk he preferred to stand and eat grass and vomit more. His poops would be runny, and then diarrhea. Sometimes his vomit would include food and other times it would be white or yellow bile. After vomiting, he would sulk and hide. Each time I became stressed and concerned that he might be in pain or that this was a sign of a serious health problem. After every instance he would go back to the veterinarian. Each time, they ran tests to rule out serious and contagious diseases. Each time the tests came back with clean results. I would hear a diagnosis of: "we're not sure, or he has a "sensitive stomach." And each time I would be given a new oral medication and new prescription foods with feeding instructions which included giving him human Pepcid tablets. The prescription foods and medicine would last a few weeks and then the bouts of vomiting and diarrhea would start up again and back to the veterinarian's office. The shelter was concerned about Tigger's health and continued to support whatever recommendation was given by the veterinarians.

> **I'd like to add a big note here,** that not all dogs in the shelters have digestive or other problems. I've heard so many people cite the myth that shelter cats and dogs are damaged goods and come with physical and psychological problems. This myth is far from the truth. There is no guarantee that any human or animal will be in perfect form and health for their entire life. One friend shared with me that his pure bred dog, from a long line of show dogs, costs him hundreds of dollars each month in allergy medications. You will read in the chapter "*How much is that Doggie in the Window*", that Dina bought a dog that she thought was coming from a reputable breeder, and ended up spending thousands on his health care. Several of my friends who have adopted rescue cats and dogs are enjoying these companions with only the costs of regular care. The love they receive in return is priceless.

Shortly after bringing him home as a foster, Tigger quickly claimed real estate in my heart so I knew I would be the one to eventually adopt him. Besides he also had a housemate cat *(see story: "An Unexpected Addition to the Family")* who were great play buddies, and I wouldn't want to separate them. Fortunately, I became a foster parent failure and was permitted to adopt him.

After the adoption papers were signed, I started to investigate what food options were available. Tigger had been on so many varieties of prescription foods, it was difficult to tell if any of them actually helped him. Since none of the test results indicated anything medically wrong with him, I wondered if he could be allergic to the food. Maybe his digestive system was intolerant of some of the ingredients. I know that when I eat a lot of junk food, or low nutrient foods that I begin to feel less than my best. Too much sugar makes me nauseous and when I don't eat enough protein I feel weaker than usual. I researched various dog diets and began by introducing him to a more natural diet.

There are several proponents to animals eating a raw diet. I attempted to give Tigger raw foods; however, regardless of what type, how small the portion or how slowly I added raw to his diet, he vomited every time he ate it. It seemed clear that his digestive system couldn't tolerate raw foods, so I continued to seek other solutions.

All the while, I talked to other dog persons. Through a friend I met a woman whose service-dog companion had once shown the same symptoms. We shared stories with each other about the struggles and concerns; and our quest to find a healthy food solution for our four legged friends. After our conversation, I visited the local holistic dog food store and purchased the same foods and probiotics she was using. I transitioned Tigger to a freeze dried food with added cooked protein, the probiotic power and a few drops of Rescue Remedy. He loves broiled chicken breast. Very quickly it appeared that his digestive system seemed to accept the chicken mixed with the freeze dried food mixture.

It's been a couple of years now that Tigger has been eating this food with a few additions. I have since added another holistic canned protein food and alternate the type of fresh lightly cooked protein. Coconut Oil has also been added to the mix. Several medical articles from veterinarians, nutritionists and medicals doctors report various health benefits of Coconut Oil. It seems to have helped Tigger as well. He put on two pounds, which the veterinarian says is his best healthy weight. His coat is naturally shiny and he no longer has flatulence. Previously his gas attacks could clear the room. Since I changed his food to holistic and natural foods, we have not had to spend time and money at the veterinarian because of digestive issues. I have also seen that even though most people were telling me that dogs should only be fed twice a day, Tigger seems to feel better when I include a small meal mid-day. Since no feeding program is universal, being mindful of Tigger's reactions to foods and feeding schedule, has been a solution that seems to have relieved the stress for both of us.

A number of my friends prepare special holistic and healthy recipes for their cats and dog companions. After her cat quit eating his regular food, one friend scoured the Internet and found a holistic recipe with balanced nutrients that also mimicked the wild food her cat companion may have caught in the wild when he was feral (i.e. rodents.) It was a healthy mixture of oats, fresh beef, ground bone (from the grocer), specific fats, fiber, and other supplements. She said it smelled good when she cooked it, and since it was all natural ingredients, admitted to tasting it once. It was tasty. Her cat agreed and ate this specially prepared food, put on a couple of needed pounds and rewarded his guardian with loud purrs and leg rubs.

It's important to make sure your animal companion will like and actually eat the food you provide. Even the healthiest balanced meal is of no value, if it's not consumed. My neighbor Carrie, cooks a special recipe for her elder dog, Bobby. Each week she cooks a batch of turkey or beef, mixed with special vitamins and a variety of vegetables. She refrigerates the mixture, and each day after heating a small portion back to room temperature, puts it in Bobby's meal dish. Someone told her that cooked green peas were healthy for dogs because they have good nutrients that support canine bone health, so she always adds them to the mixture, even though Bobby doesn't appear to like them. Maybe he eats a few, however, when he is finished eating and walks away, he leaves behind a neat row of peas on the floor beside his dish.

An old adage "at least you've got your health", said when someone is lamenting about problems in their lives, indicates the importance we place on our good health. Many researchers believe that what we eat has an effect on our health and can actually be a cause of serious illnesses - such as type2 diabetes, obesity, heart disease, stroke and certain cancers. The same is true for our cats and dogs. Being unhealthy, either human or animal, is not only expensive, it robs us of the good quality of life. Read the labels of the foods your buy. Look for companies that offer wholesome natural food products.

Watch your animal companions for their reactions and their body changes in response to certain foods. Consult with a nutritionist or take time to research good nutrition in books and on the internet. When a problem appears, i.e.: personality changes, changes in poop, vomiting, extreme or sudden weight gain/loss etc.; don't hesitate - visit your trusted veterinarian or animal naturopath and find a solution. 8

Pet food recalls:
http://www.accessdata.fda.gov/scripts/newpetfoodrecalls

"Purring is an automatic safety valve device for dealing with happiness overflow"

- Original Author unverified

Dangerous Foods

Some foods, spices and chemicals can post pose hazards for cats & dogs. Some of the top most dangerous foods include:

Alcoholic beverages- all types
Can cause intoxication, coma, and death.

Avocado
The leaves, seeds, fruit, and bark contain persin, which can cause vomiting and diarrhea. Excessive vomiting and diarrhea can cause dehydration which could lead to death.

Bones from fish, poultry, or cooked bones from other meat sources
Can cause obstruction or laceration of the digestive system. These bones can break off in slivers and puncture the esophagus.

Dogs should not eat Cat food
Cat food is generally too high in protein and fats. Too much fat in a dogs diet can cause pancreatitis, which can be deadly.

Dogs should not eat Cat food

Dog food does not have enough nutrients for Cats. A steady diet of dog food can cause your cat to be severely malnourished.

Chocolate, coffee, tea, and other caffeine

Any beverage containing caffeine can cause a dog's heart to race, sometimes causing seizures.

Grapes and raisins

Contain an unknown toxin, which can damage the kidneys.

Human vitamin supplements containing iron.

Can damage the lining of the digestive system and be toxic to the other organs including the liver and kidneys.

Marijuana

Can depress the nervous system, cause vomiting, and changes in the heart rate.

Milk and other dairy products

Even though many cartoons show a cat lapping a saucer of milk, some adult dogs and cats may develop diarrhea if given large amounts of dairy products.

Moldy or spoiled food, garbage

It's a myth that domesticated animals can eat anything. Garbage can contain multiple toxins which can cause illness and even death.

Mushrooms

The toxins can cause shock, and result in death. This includes the wild mushrooms growing in your yard.

Onions garlic (raw, cooked, or powder)

Contains thiosulphate, which is toxic. Cats are more susceptible than dogs. Yes, you will read these ingredients on certain cat and dog food products. According to various manufacturers, the small amounts used have not been indicated as creating problems. Various recipes include adding powdered garlic. Be very careful when adding garlic to your animal companion's diet. Be prepared to recognize the first sign of problems. Raw garlic and onions are always a problem, including the partially cooked ones in human menus.

Pits from peaches and plums

Can cause obstruction of the digestive tract.

Salt

If eaten in large quantities it may lead to electrolyte imbalances.

String

Can become trapped in the digestive system. *(See chapter "Kitten Proofing")*

Tobacco

Contains nicotine. If ingested it can effects the digestive and nervous systems. Can result in rapid heartbeat, collapse, coma, and death. Studies indicate that second hand smoke is harmful to humans. It is also harmful to animals. If they inhale second hand smoke. it can cause rapid heartbeat, breathing difficulties, bronchial spasms, cancers and death.

Xylitol (artificial sweetener used in many diet products and candies)

Can cause very low blood sugar, which can result in vomiting, weakness and collapse. In high doses can cause liver failure.

Acetaminophen (Tylenol), Ibuprofen (Advil/Motrin, etc.), Amphetamines (Medications)

Human pain relievers and medications can be toxic.

More links to resources on toxic foods can be found on the Stress Out for Cats and Dogs website.

Besides certain foods being poisonous to cats and dogs, certain flowers and plants can also be toxic. When Merlin was a kitten, he had an interest in chewing on my plants. Quick research identified which plants in my home would be deadly to him. They were immediately removed. He was then given several small pots of cat grass to nibble instead. A detailed list of poisonous plants can be found at: http://www.petpoisonhelpline.com/poisons

Bugs and insects are something else to be aware of. Bee stings are rarely lethal unless your cat or dog has an allergic reaction which would then require veterinary care. Mosquito bites are possibly the most common insect bite to animals. Heartworm is carried by mosquitoes and is deadly. (See chapter on Heartworm) Fleas and ticks are other common parasites. Fleas can cause anemia, tapeworms, allergies and skin infections from constant scratching. Each year, thousands of cats and dogs become infected with serious diseases, anemia or paralysis caused by ticks. Ticks and fleas can be worse from one area to another and can vary seasonally and from year to year. Educate yourself on your area's flea and tick seasons. Examine your cat and dog carefully after a walk or play time outside. To find fleas look for areas that appear to have dried blood, or small black dots which look like dirty spots. Watch where your animal companion is biting or constantly scratching themself or areas where they are losing fur. To search for ticks, run your hands all over the body, paying close attention to the ears neck, skin folds and other crevices. You may prefer to wear latex gloves. The ASPCA offers detailed instructions for removing ticks on their website.[15]

Rats. In some areas rats are a constant problem. Rat poison is lethal to all animals. If your cat or dog kills, bites into or ingests a rat which has eaten rat poison, they will poisoned as well. Some people belief that something poisonous will make your cat or dog vomit. That is not true. Rat poisons can be fatal even in small amounts. Some gardeners and home owners place rat poison in their gardens, and unsuspecting people allow their dogs to roam and sniff that area. One year we had incidences of several dogs eating rat poison that someone threw into a park area to kill rodents. It was after the sudden death of a few dogs before someone discovered the reason. To be safe, know what rat poison looks like; don't put any in your home or yard that is accessible by your animals; avoid bushes and grassy areas where rats might live or hide; keep any of your chemicals locked safely away.

Something as beautiful as a butterfly can also be deadly. Monarch butterflies feed on milkweed which is poisonous to Cats and Dogs. If they eat a Monarch butterfly, they could be poisoned by what the butterfly had eaten.

Our animal companions rely upon us to keep them safe and healthy. If you suspect your cat or dog has eaten something toxic, please note the amount ingested, their reactions and contact your veterinarian or the ASPCA Animal Poison Control Center at (888) 426-4435.

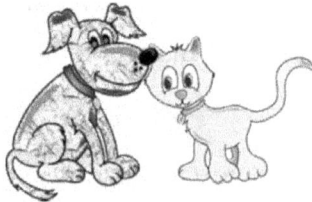

Natural Healing

By Sue Heldenbrand

I had a dog named Duchess who was a mixed German Shepard and Belgian Malinois. Many of these large breed dogs tend to get hip displacement which causes them pain. Duchess was no exception. During her early life, she was very energetic and protective of her turf. But as the years started to add on, the discomfort in her hip area began to show. I would put her inside my house during the night and let her out in the morning. She started to gradually have trouble getting up. Using an energetic based modality, I would work on releasing the pain in that area. I would work on the area for a few minutes and then stop. She would raise her paw at me, letting me know that she wanted more. After a few more minutes of doing energy work on her, she would then get up and was ready to go outside. This continued for many years and I helped her age with less pain and discomfort.

See "About the Authors" section to learn more about Sue Heldenbrand.

"Dogs are the leaders of the planet.
If you see two life forms, one of them is making a poop,
the other one's carrying it for him,
who would you assume is in charge."
~ Jerry Seinfeld

Shadrach
the Teacher Dog

By Kim Bloomer, V.N.D.

Shadrach appeared healthy, although things were changing and I couldn't help but notice. I had continued with a traditional approach to his care at first, but Shadrach wasn't going to allow me to stay there.

I took him to the vet to have his anal sacs checked because the horrible familiar smell from my days in veterinary medicine was very evident to me. Unfortunately he had impacted sacs, which had to be drained, and he was put on some meds to help him heal. I had never had to clean out the anal sacs while I worked at the veterinary clinic, so I asked Shadrach's current vet to show me how to do it, which he gladly did. Shadrach had been neutered and vaccinated elsewhere, so it was his first time to be seen at this particular clinic.

Unfortunately it wouldn't be long before we were back again, because Shadrach contracted Bordatella, more commonly known as kennel cough. One of his "girlfriends" from the park, Kuma, had gotten the same disease at the groomer's. It's interesting to note that both Shadrach and Kuma had received the standard vaccine against kennel cough and yet they both contracted the illness. This is caused by a virus similar to the common cold in humans, but with a deep, hacking cough. It is conventionally treated with antibiotics. We all know that antibiotics are not effective against viruses, so why they are prescribed as the standard medication makes no sense to me today. However, at that time I trustingly put Shadrach through two months of antibiotic treatment, which ultimately caused his immune system to decline severely (the antibiotics killed all the GOOD immune supportive bacteria along with the bad and had no effect whatsoever on the viruses they were prescribed for). Rest, plenty of purified water, a raw diet (which he wasn't getting YET), colloidal silver, PRObiotics, enzymes and colostrum would have been not only a better protocol to follow, but a healing and immune system building one as well. Unfortunately I had not yet learned all of that.

At the same time I kept trying to find some type of kibble that he would readily eat. I was mystified why a formerly starved dog was not interested in eating all this "good" food. So began my quest into natural animal health. I started researching food, and then began adding cooked meats, veggies and other "junk" into the food I was giving him. Shadrach would methodically pick out the meat and leave the rest. Eventually, after I tried everything I could think of to get him to eat his veggies AND kibble, I discovered that that was not what a carnivore was meant to eat. Shadrach had been trying to tell me this all along. The cooking part mattered little (although he does prefer a little warmth to his food), reminding me of what Golum said to one of the Hobbits in a "Lord of the Rings" movie... Sam, a rotund young Hobbit, was cooking a nice pot of rabbit stew and Golum screeched in a tantrum, "What are you doing to it, you fat, stupid Hobbit! I like it raw and still wiggling!" Most dogs will do just fi ne with pure raw meat and bones, cold or otherwise.

The final incident to send me headlong into the promotion of natural animal health happened late one night. We'd noticed some strangely parallel strips of missing hair along each side of Shadrach's body, and I took him to his vet to see what was going on. The vet did skin scrapes and determined the cause to be "idiopathic" – which translated means he had no idea what it was. So he did what all doctors and veterinarians apparently do when the diagnosis is determined to be "idiopathic": he prescribed topical and internal antibiotics. Sometimes they will also include steroids. I could go off on a tangent here about the logic behind this treatment, but I'll spare you the tirade because at that time I was as ignorant of the facts as are those in the veterinary profession who have not seen the light yet.

I began Shadrach's course of topical and internal antibiotics immediately, but by the following day he was vomiting off and on, so his vet advised we discontinue the internal antibiotics and continue using the topical ones only. I went to bed early that night, totally exhausted, but about two hours later Donnie roused me from a dead sleep to say that Shadrach was heaving and hacking as though he couldn't breathe. Within minutes I was dressed and we were off to the emergency animal clinic.

I remember Donnie asking me if I wanted a hat - I thought it was because of the cold winter air - and I said, "NO, let's just go!" I later discovered it was because I'd not brushed my sleep-messed hair and Donnie was doing his best to be subtle about it. No doubt I resembled Cruella de Vil from the movie, 101 Dalmatians! When we arrived I immediately informed the vet I was a former vet assistant and wanted to "get to the nitty gritty" of what was going on with Shadrach right away. In my panic, I feared it was torsion (the digestive illness seen dogs such as Great Danes), so she began quoting the exorbitant costs of its treatment, and I finally had to ask her to please just determine what was wrong first! X-rays were taken, and it was apparent that Shadrach had aspirated vomit into his lungs, causing pneumonia. (MY personal diagnosis was a drug-induced pneumonia due to his reaction to the antibiotics that brought it all on in the first place!) We were advised to leave Shadrach with them until morning...or rather told to leave him there! I have since learned that considering the fact that he is our dog, we make the demands, and not the health care practitioners, especially since we're the ones who pay the bill!

We hardly slept that night and were back at the clinic door at 8 AM. All I could think about was what Shadrach must have felt when we walked off and left him there the night before. Because of the abuse he had previously suffered before he came to us, we had a natural tendency to want to shelter him. Several hundred dollars later we got him back, sicker than ever. And what sent me "over the edge" was the fact that he had poop all over his backside and no one there had even bothered to clean him up, and he also had a catheter in his hind leg with the bandage so tight that his leg had swollen up to twice its normal size! I immediately took him to our regular vet, and he too was furious at the treatment Shadrach had received at the emergency clinic. He was also very apologetic that Shadrach had been put through so much.

Nothing could calm my anger at the time, although I now feel I might have more appropriately directed the majority of it at myself for not being better informed and aware of my available choices for him. The emergency clinic had also given poor Shadrach even MORE antibiotics, another thing which made little sense to me, but which I permitted anyway. Immediately after this horrendous episode, I began my mission to find out all I could about natural animal health and to see to it that Shadrach never had to endure anything like that again. Donnie figured out that the skin "disorder" was Shadrach's allergic response to the new paint in our house. He always leans up against our walls, so by keeping him from doing that his skin healed. We also used the ointment and animal shampoo by Young Living that a new online friend sent to me free of charge. And at that point my "journey" truly began in earnest. I was on a mission to share what I knew with the rest of the world. I began blogging and writing about natural animal health. I went back to school, earned my degrees, and I'm now studying for a degree as doctor of naturopathy in human health.

I've learned so much about the harm we can cause our animals by using what we thought was helping them. Vaccines, processed food, topical flea and tick medicines, and even the internal medicines for heartworm and parasites can do grave, long-term damage to animals. I realize that many people (laymen and professionals alike) will vehemently disagree with me, but that's okay because I have learned the truth. I stepped out of my comfort zone because of one stubborn, willful and absolutely wonderful dog by the name of Shadrach. Previously Shadrach would try and run from me whenever I attempted to apply the topical flea and tick control. And then as soon as I had applied it he would be rolling in the grass trying to rub it off , then in the dirt, and then back to the grass, doing his best to get that junk off of himself. You would have thought I'd get at least a clue from the package directions, which stated that gloves should be worn when applying. Whatever we put ON our animals eventually goes INTO them, thus burdening and taxing the liver and other filtration organs such as the skin, lungs, kidneys, etc.

Even though I was earning my degrees and receiving my education, Shadrach still had some lessons of his own to teach me. One morning he accidentally slid down into a cement arroyo constructed by the city to contain the fast-flowing water runoff s so frequent during our thunderstorms. Donnie told me Shadrach slid sideways and arrived home with a few scrapes and bruises in addition to a bruised ego. I took care of his topical scrapes with some of the natural ointment and essential oils I use, thinking that he was okay.

A few months later I discovered I was wrong about my treatment. First he had a pancreatic attack - which I addressed and pulled him through using an entirely natural protocol. And then he started walking with his front right paw knuckling over which led me to an animal chiropractor who greatly helped him. Then, to rule out any fractures, I had him x-rayed by his regular vet (although he has since been

146

seen by a holistic vet as well), who discovered that Shadrach had a few arthritic changes in his elbow (and now his hips), which I control with supplements rather than pharmaceuticals. All in all, I continue to keep him healthy with occasional treatments by the animal chiropractor and the use of essential oils, herbs, supplements, and massage. For the most part I generally monitor and take care of his health issues myself. He has not been on any form of drugs or medications since that awful visit to the emergency animal clinic.

Shadrach has been my "teacher dog" for almost ten years, and he continues to educate me. He's the reason I went back to school, why I blog and write, why I do an online radio show, and why I now help other pet owners be empowered with the knowledge they need to care for their animals according to God's provision in nature.

See "About the Authors" section to learn more about Dr. Kim Bloomer.

The Message in Poop

By Leslie May

I have two adorable dogs, Mickey and Luke. Like many people I have relied on the ease of a doggie door and a fenced back yard for my dog's potty needs. We have a large backyard and our gardener cleans up all the droppings each week. I seldom get my hands dirty when it comes to my dogs.

Both of my dogs seem to love the park and the new adventures on the trails near our home, and even though I kept them on leashes, they explore, sniff, and water every leaf, twig and blade of grass along the way.

The only problem was when they would poop. The most nauseating thing to me is cleaning up my dog's poop. I had no problem changing very messy baby diapers, but I need plastic gloves to clean up after my dogs.

I know it's the law in my area and I've heard the preaching around the health hazards of left behind poop, but that didn't make any difference to me for a long time. I always carried bags with me, just in case - just in case someone else saw my dogs poop and expected me to clean it up. For a while I would say I ran out of bags until I got an earful from another dog owner about being responsible and always prepared. So I'd carry bags, but when I'd see my dogs circling for a squat I would turn my back and pretend I didn't see what happened. Then I'd walk away from quickly from the scene. It was much later that I learned that even when I thought I wasn't seen, that people across the park had watched my dog poop and my pretend unawareness. I was actually talked about as one of **those** people. That was embarrassing to hear I had such a reputation.

Friends would send me articles and links and I would give the excuse that I didn't have time to read the emails. What I did learn, even when I was trying not to, was that even though wild animal poop may biodegrade back into the soil, dog poop is not a fertilizer. We feed our dogs food that's very different from the food wild animals eat. Dog poop can attract certain insects that carry disease contain harmful organisms like E. coli, giardia, salmonella and worms in dogs. Poop from sick dogs is how some dogs get sick from being around these dogs. Some poop left behind gets smashed into the grass or ground and may appear to disappear and be gone, but walking across that area or kids playing on it can be enough to pick up the bacteria. Sprinklers can wash away much of this bacteria from a park or backyard lawn, but in many places, it becomes part of the groundwater that then becomes the water that we get from our taps. In my area of San Diego, California, the Environmental Protection Agency estimated that 2-3 days' worth of poop from 100 dogs would contribute enough bacteria to temporarily close a 20 miles stretch of beach. This became a reality for us in the year 2000 when one of our dog beaches was closed 125 times to surfers and swimmers. It seems sad that dog owners, like me, were the cause of this problem, especially when this beach has dog baggie stations and receptacles right there in plain sight. Unfortunately, even hearing this at the time didn't change my lazy behavior. It took something more personal to me

A few months ago I decided my dogs and I needed more outside time together. Now I look at this as an Angel intervention to show me I needed to pay attention to something. We have beautiful trails near our home so the walks can be breathtaking. This day I felt like talking my dogs for a walk on one of these trails.

Halfway through our second walk I discovered something that caused me concern. When I glanced over and saw one of my dogs, Mickey, taking his poop, I noticed he had severe diarrhea. His personality was still as loving as usual, so I first thought it was just a temporary sign of indigestion. But Mickey seemed to get worse as we walked, stopping frequently and sitting down (something new). He still seemed to respond normally with his tail wagging when I could coax him to come to me. But something was definitely not right. I called the veterinarian and we abandoned our walk in the park, went right over.

Good thing we did. After several tests, the verdict was that Mickey had pancreatitis, a very serious and sometimes fatal condition. He was going to need to stay a few days at the vet's office for fluids, medication and more tests. As the veterinarian explained the seriousness of the diagnosis, she also questioned me as to when I first observed the symptoms.

I'd really only seen his diarrhea that one day, but the vet said he had been suffering for a while. Pancreatitis can be painful. So my sweet dog had been suffering and I didn't know. The severity of Mickey's condition indicated that he had been suffering longer than just this one day. He is such a well behaved dog, and since his personality *seemed* normal, I had no suspicion that anything might be wrong until I saw the diarrhea.

I was so sad leaving Mickey at the veterinarian and returning home with only one dog, Duncan. When I returned home, I decided to visit their potty area in the back yard. In several spots, I discovered what appeared to be diarrhea, and some had what looked like dried blood.

I hadn't seen the early signs. I wasn't around when my dogs use the yard, and I don't do the cleanup.. On top of that, I was negligent in watching and picking up their poop when we were away from home, I felt so guilty. I needed to make some changes.

I now schedule walks at least three times a week with my dogs and I pay closer attention to any change in their behavior. Looking back I can remember small changes in Mickey's behavior that I didn't consider significant at the time. Now I know differently. I'm also watching my dogs a little more often when they are in the back yard, and my gardener has been instructed to tell me if any of my dogs poop appears suspicious.

I know it was an Angel that got me out of the chair and onto that trail with my dogs that day. That same Angel made me look at Mickey at just that right time. If I hadn't taken that walk with Duncan and Mickey, the result might have been different, and I would be wondering (and feeling terrible) when Mickey would have gotten sicker, or worse. Pancreatitis can be fatal.

I am now paying closer attention to what they eat. I was told by the Vet that pancreatitis can be caused by too much fatty foods or an unbalanced, unhealthy diet. I used to think that dogs could eat anything and it really didn't matter. Now I feel differently. I don't eat junk food, so my dogs don't either. My friends think I'm a little extravagant, but I have seen a dog nutritionist to help me choose the best diet for my dogs.

It's still hard for me to pick up poop, but my dog's lives are worth a few minutes of me feeling yucky. It's easy to fall into lazy habits, and it does take conscious commitment to change, but my boys are worth it. I am grateful for that Angel.

Live More Like a Dog

By Eileen Gould

I have loved dogs from as far back as I could remember. My first dog was bubbles and he was a darling poodle that had curly hair. During the time I had Bubbles in Philadelphia, my mom got cancer. I remember Bubbles being a comfort; a friend I could talk too, cuddle with and cry on.

During my single years it was impossible to have a dog.
As soon as I married and had kids we got our son a Cocker Spaniel named Billie. Billie was part of our family, and lived to be 17. He is now buried in a monument in my back yard. Now, I have Emma, a white lab, and Baxter a French Bulldog.

I cook them chicken everyday. I am careful to not give them bones in the chicken. I season it carefully. I also brush their teeth and wipe their butt. My kids think I am overdoing it and probably you do too.

What I have found is that these four- legged children of mine, know my moods, know my feelings and know me probably better than my family. I can talk to them and find empathy, and love. I can lay with them and find peace, and get through hard times just looking in their eyes. Perhaps, if you are an animal lover you know exactly how I feel.

If we lived life more like a dog, and just could be here now, I believe it would be a happier world.

"Dogs are our link to paradise.
They don't know evil or jealousy or discontent.
To sit with a dog on a hillside on a glorious afternoon
is to be back in Eden, where doing nothing
was not boring, it was peace."
~ Milan Kundera

SAFETY

"The soul is the same in all living creatures,
although the body of each is different."
~ Hippocrates

Kitten Safety

"There is no more intrepid explorer than a kitten."

~ Jules Champfleury

As soon as Merlin came to live in my home I had to re-learn that nothing was safe in my house and all of my secrets would soon be discovered. Merlin is the first kitten I've had in my home for over 15 years. My previous cat companion, Lancelot, was well beyond his kitten behavior for so many years, that I'd forgotten how inquisitive a kitten can be. After all my decorating efforts to make my home reflect my personality, Merlin made sure his presence was immediately known, and he's now the master of my decor.

In the beginning, I had to put away my delicate crystal and china trinkets and purchase a new batch of earthquake hold for other items. A friend stated that kitten proofing is just like baby proofing a home. I must partially disagree. Although the commitment to safety is similar, as far as I know, babies don't move at lightning speed from one point to another. Nor do they leap from the floor to the top shelf of the bookcase in one smooth move. It never ceases to amaze me how Merlin can surefootedly walk across the smallest ledge and disturb nothing. Then decide that he must get into the one-half inch space between a something and the wall; sending the object toppling to the floor. One such object was a vase holding Chinese fortune plants and filled with water. After he pushed his little body between the vase and the wall, the vase fortunately (?) landed in my open briefcase below and not all over the tile floor. The briefcase kept the vase from breaking, but it was never the same.

My home is filled with growing plants. I love the living green inside, and so does Merlin. At first, many smaller plants were moved to higher locations. When I did this, I had a memory lapse about cats ability to jump. Merlin seemed to like to chomp on certain leaves and dig in the soil. With over 300 plants toxic to cats, I've had to educate myself and made sure that none of these were inside my home. When I first took Merlin to the Veterinarian after rescuing him, he stated that Merlin appeared to have been on the street for a while. So using dirt as his bathroom would be something he was previously accustomed to and I certainly didn't want him to mistake any of these plants for a litter box.

Many people use spray bottles and loud noises to startle a cat and attempt to train their behavior. I've read that these methods only stop the cat from whatever they are doing, when you are present but doesn't help to change the undesired behavior when you aren't home or aren't looking, such as in the night. The cats relate the noise or wetness to the guardian who is holding the sprayer or noise maker, instead of to their own behavior. I wanted something more natural and loving. There are several liquid and spray deterrent products on the marketplace as well. However, after reading their ingredient labels and getting a whiff of the smell, these didn't appear to be the non-toxic, healthy solution I was seeking for my home.

To attempt to keep Merlin out of the plants, I started by placing little stakes in the pots surrounding the plants, making a vertical type of fence. Merlin chewed on the stakes and let himself through. So, that didn't work. Then, I took clear packaging tape and put it sticky side out. That kept him from climbing on the larger pots, and it's sooo attractive to my decor. Not to mention how many times I caught my clothing the tape as I passed by.

A friend suggested orange peels and coffee grounds. Allegedly, cats don't like the smell of citrus. It appears Merlin is one of those cats. I placed the orange peels around the outer edge of the pot, and zested some of the peel into water and sprayed the leaves. The coffee grounds are sprinkled over the top of the soil. Coffee grounds are also a natural air freshener, so that is an added bonus. Another friend suggested aquarium gravel, as cats don't necessarily like the feel of the uneven edges under their paws. For those plants with a larger soil surface area I added natural gravel as well.

After only a week, Merlin moved onto other investigations around the house and my safe-for-cats-and-dogs plants were left alone to flourish, for a while. It was then that I introduced cat grass. He loves it and started to choose the cat grass over my plants. Even now, whenever there is cat grass available to him, he stays away from my plants. It can be costly to continue to buy at the store, so I now buy the seeds and plant them in cute pots. The seeds only take a few days to grow and when timed appropriately, Merlin always has a fresh growth to nibble.

My kitchen was soon identified as another area I needed to be mindful of Merlin. Anytime I go to the kitchen, he follows. Even though he doesn't always get food, I believe he knows it's there and remains ever hopeful. I've seen him on top of the refrigerator which I believe he gets to by first jumping on the counter. Now, before doing anything in the kitchen I wash the counter tops with vinegar, just in case he used them during the night. I'm not bothered by Merlin on the one countertop near the refrigerator. I can always wash the small area, however, I want him to stay away from the stove; so I use a product that was recommended by a cat behaviorist's website. It's a motion detection device that sends a quick burst of air towards Merlin when he gets within 3 feet of where I don't want him to be. I use this at night or when I'm not home. I only bought one because they are a bit costly and I use it for the kitchen counter.

When I'm cooking I am extra mindful of Merlin. Before I start my preparations, I create a safe place for Merlin. He has a specially placed chair right outside the kitchen. My kitchen is small, so the chair is actually approximately 6 feet away from me. The chair is so he can be close enough to observe and be out of harm's way. When he approaches the kitchen when I'm cooking I coax him to the chair. When he sits on the chair he gets a treat and a few scratches behind the ear. Anytime he gets down and starts to enter the kitchen while I'm cooking, I repeat the coaxing and the attention. The treats and scratches alternate, because I don't want him addicted to always getting treats. Sometimes an ear scratch or nose nudge is enough. Yes, this does require me to wash my hand a few more times while I'm cooking, however, it's easier than trying to shoo him out, or picking him up and moving him out. Consistency is the key. If the chair is not present, he waltzes into the kitchen. A minute to place a chair saves me the stress of always looking for him underfoot or attempting to stop him mid-air in a jump. Even though I take the time to keep him out of the kitchen when I'm cooking, I still take additional precautions when I'm finished cooking and taking the time to eat my meal. All pots and pans have lids on them and hot burners are covered with a pot lid or similar to prevent kitten feet from touching the hot area. I also place the motion detector air sprayer device back in its place. I had always assumed that a kitten would instinctively know when a surface was hot and to avoid it. I learned differently when a friend shared that her new kitten jumped up and landed on her hot stove, and in its attempt to get away from the area, knocked over a bowl of hot gravy on itself and the floor. A little time can save a lot of pain and extra cleanup.

I learned the hard way the importance of providing appropriate play toys for my feline companions. Shoestrings, cord and thread can be deadly. When Lancelot first came to live with me he bought a sister, Ariel with him. He was all white and she was mostly black, except for a tiny white mark on her chin and the toes on one paw. I lovingly said that it looked like she put her paw in the milk and still had drops on her chin. Ariel was beautiful and very playful. As a kitten she could chase anything that moved and would continue to attack it long after she had captured it. I would use the shoestrings from my workout shoes as a toy and afterwards it appeared that she enjoyed "killing" my shoes and the strings.

One morning when cleaning her litter box, I noticed a small piece of shoestring next to her poop. I thought that perhaps she had pooped on top of a piece of string that she had carried into her litter box. Later that morning I heard her meow when she left the litter box and I saw what looked like a piece of string coming out of her anus. She ran away from me. Then sat down and proceeded to have dry heaves and convulsions. With help, I got her into a carrier and to the veterinarian. After tests and x-rays, it was determined that she had swallowed a piece of shoelace and it was lodged in her intestine. Surgery was required to remove it, after which the veterinarian wanted to keep her a couple of days for observation. She never came home. The veterinarian called to tell me that her little heart gave out from the stress of the blocked intestine, the convulsions and the surgery. I was devastated and feeling guilty. Ariel had died from a game I had started with her. Later I would learn from other people that shoelaces are inappropriate; but at the time I didn't know. Both Lancelot and I grieved over the loss of Ariel for a long time.

Merlin is not allowed in the closet next to my shoes. I don't taunt him with shoestrings or loose cord of any kind. All his toys are too big to swallow; and if they get overly shredded from his active play, they are replaced. His favorite toys are empty bags of any kind, crumpled paper under my desk, the dog's squeaky toys and something called DaBird, which has feathers on a cord at the end of a stick. DaBird is only out when I using it to play with him. He can catch it and hide it during play, but when our playtime is over, it gets put away. Some cats are okay around this type of toy and wouldn't chew on it after play. With a dog in the house who also likes to chew on things, this toy is too much of a temptation to be chewed in smaller pieces, which then have the potential of being swallowed.

Merlin's all-time favorite plaything is Tigger. From behind a corner or under a piece of furniture he will leap out and attack. They rough and tumble; taking turns who's chasing who. They seem to know the limits and no blood is ever drawn. Merlin appears to keep his claws in during play. I keep them trimmed just in case. The shelter where I volunteered recommended that we take time to lightly massage the cat's paws and toes. By doing this, the cats were more accepting when someone was holding their paw and clipping their nails. I followed that practice with Merlin, so I can keep his nail trimmed, and Tigger and my skin a little safer from scratches. Not all dogs and cats can get along and play together as well as these two. I think it's partially because they came into my home within months of each other and grew up together. Watching animals play is free entertainment and a great stress relief.

Being aware of my animal companion's personalities and their tendency to chew on things makes it important for me to be aware of what is in my home and any potential hazards. Breakable items are either packed up for now, or secured with earthquake hold. Plants are both cat and dog friendly or they are gone. Toys are appropriate for both Merlin's personality and Tigger's possessiveness. If Merlin is playing with it,

Tigger wants it, too. Tiny balls that Merlin might chase could potentially get caught in Tigger's throat if he swallowed them.

My friends accuse me of being overly protective. We've laughed while they tell me they believe I would keep them in a safety bubble if I could. After losing one devoted precious black kitten to not knowing how dangerous a piece of string could be, I am willing to be overly cautious and teased about it. I am becoming well trained and educated on what is safe for the animal companions that depend on me.

"My mother told me cats drink out of the toilet

because the water is cold in there.

And I'm like: How did my mother know that?"

~ Wendy Liebman

Holiday Safety

Safety is important every day; however certain holidays bring extra needs for safety measures.

During any holiday celebration:

NO Alcohol. I've heard of people who think it's funny to give their dog or cat companion "just a little" and then laugh at their drunken behavior. Alcoholic beverages are toxic to animals and should never be given to them at any time.

Leftovers. Leftover chicken and turkey can contain dangerous bones which could splinter when being chewed or swallowed. Ham is high in fat. If you are going to feed your animals leftovers, check extra carefully for bones and make sure the cooking recipe was free of spices toxic to animals *(ie: nutmeg, onion, etc. See chapter Dangerous Foods)* One cause of pancreatitis can be a sudden excess of a fat as in the holiday turkey and ham leftovers. If you feed table scraps that you know are safe, it's best to put the food in their regular bowl. Feeding your dog directly from the table can result in bad manners and begging.

Valentine's Day:
Flowers and Candy. Many types of plants found in bouquets are harmful to dogs and cats if they are ingested. A detailed list of poisonous plants can be found at:
http://www.petpoisonhelpline.com/poisons

Do not share your chocolate with your furry friends. It can cause vomiting, diarrhea, hyperactivity, abnormal heart rhythm, tremors and seizures, and in severe cases, chocolate poisoning can be fatal.

Easter:
Colorful fake grass may look appetizing and even fun to your animal friends, but it could cause them to choke or obstruct their intestines if ingested. Small toys and other plastic items, if swallowed, can cause your pet to choke or even damage their intestinal tracts.

4th July:
Fireworks can scare your pets making them run off, or cause serious injuries if detonated near them. Many formulations are also toxic if ingested.

If your pets are excitable by loud noises even when at home, put them in a room or crate while you are out so they feel safe.

Halloween:
It's that time of year again where all sorts of goblins and witches wander the street in search of things sweet. Some of these are two legged and many are accompanied by their four legged friends. This is also the time you front door will be

opened again and again during the evening. This can increase the chances of your dogs and cats running out. Keep an eye on their whereabouts, or better yet, keep them safe in another room away from the front door.

Safety is important to both humans and animals. Some people include their animal companions in their costumes; other cats and dogs can be seen wandering alone hoping for a handout. (*See reminder about chocolate.*)

Reconsider if you are planning on taking your dog out trick or treating. (*See chapter "Jades Halloween Adventure"*) If you do, be extra diligent in watching your surroundings and keep them on a shorter than usual leash. Make sure they have their tags on and something reflective helps them to be seen. People are accustomed to seeing children; they can easily overlook a small dog walking beside you. If you do take your pet out wearing a costume, make sure it fits well enough so they can walk, have clear field of vision, and that they are comfortable in it. If they struggle to get it off, or whine while wearing it - it is a sign they don't like it, no matter how cute you think they look. Make sure there are no little pieces they can chew on and swallow. Ties and ribbons can pull loose and get caught around their necks or legs causing them to trip. Some plastic costumes hold in your dog's body heat and can make them pant harder than usual. Make sure your dog is well ventilated and well hydrated. Be prepared to stop when they need a potty break and remember to take potty bags. No one wants to bring home the unwanted smelly dog poop on their feet.

Thanksgiving

Veterinarian offices and Animal Emergency Rooms are busier during the holidays treating dogs that have splintered boned in their throats and intestines. Keep them away from the Turkey until you have made sure it is free of bones and spices which are toxic to cats and dogs.

Christmas

Many holiday plants such as Christmas rose, Holly, Lilies and Mistletoe are all toxic to cats and dogs. Christmas Tree Angel hair can be irritating to the eyes and skin and if eaten could cause intestinal obstruction. Tinsel can cause choking or intestinal blockage if swallowed. Christmas tree water, stagnant tree water or water containing preservatives including ASPIRIN could result in stomach upset if ingested. It might be entertaining to watch funny videos of animals in Christmas trees, however, there's nothing funny about an animal tangled and injured by the tree, its lights or decorations. Cats will love to bat around the baubles on your tree because they move and sometimes make noise. Enough batting around can cause the decoration to fall to the floor and if glass, shatter. Tiny specs of glass can get into pet hair and feet, and if they lick themselves, can be ingested and cause trauma in their stomach and intestines.

Chanukah

Be aware of candles left burning. They may brush by and burn their fur, or get burned by the candle dripping. Cats love to jump and investigate, especially something moving, even a candle flame. Keep all burning candles in areas safe from animal intuitiveness. The high amount of fat in Hanukkah doughnuts and Latkas could be too much for safe eating for cats and dogs. Latkas contain onions which are toxic to cats and dogs. The Dreidel and other game toys can be intriguing to watch and if small enough can cause choking or intestinal blockage if swallowed. Be watchful that your children don't share their chocolate coins with your furry friends.

New Years

Decorations, food and alcohol are almost synonymous with New Year's Eve. Balloons and confetti decorations can cause your pets to choke or obstruct their intestines if ingested. Alcohol can be toxic. Drunk party revelers can trip over, fall on top of and step on small animals. The loud noises of New Year's eve can frighten them and cause them to run off. Always watch your buffet for curious dogs and guests feeding your animals from their plate. For their safety, it is best to keep them in a room away from all the activity and noise.

"Somewhere in a parallel universe, there's a giant dog carrying a little woman in her purse."

~Original author unverified

Jade's Halloween Adventure

By Bridget Clovis

Halloween has always been a night of fun when as a child I was allowed to dress up as my favorite fantasy character. I have enjoyed this tradition with my children as well with each squeal and laugh at the costumes and decorations.

As a child I used to dress up the family dog in costume as well so he could be part of my fantasy. My mother never allowed me to take him trick-or-treating with me, citing she had too many kids to keep an eye on and the dog would be happier at home. My own children have enjoyed dressing up our golden retriever, Jade, each Halloween and playing with him in costume for several hours before they were allowed to venture outside for our annual candy collecting ritual.

One year changed all this.

My 9 year old daughter, Marcie, dressed as a police officer and she wanted her "police" dog to accompany her on our route. My first reaction was to echo my mother's reasons for no dogs on the tour, but then Jade looked so cute with his official "police" vest, badge and "police" cap, and he was so well known and loved in our neighborhood that I agreed to let him go. Marcie promised she would hold tight onto Jade's leash, "because that's what the police do." Jade was leash trained since a tiny puppy to never pull. Marcie had walked him with me responsibly holding his leash several times and so I agreed he could come. Her younger brothers were Batman and Superman, so it appeared like a super quad.

Everything was fine for the first few houses. Several families had included their dogs in the costume festivities, so I was happy to show off Jade and his co-costume. Then the crowd of children starting growing larger and a little unruly at some houses. At one house there were so many children scrambling to squeeze through a gate to get the candy that was being distributed, that Jade's paws were stepped on twice. I started to hold back from the crowds and approached only houses that had the fewest visitors. I was getting concerned about Jade and all the chaos so I took his leash from Marcie. At one house, Stevie's batman cape got caught on a fence and we stopped. I put my hand through the loop in Jade's leash, wearing it like a bracelet, to give me both hands free to release Stevie's cape. Suddenly, a few teenagers dressed in black and Goth, teamed with a big black lab, came running up. Kids running everywhere was not uncommon, so I glanced at these kids and went back to Stevie. Then I heard a growl and I was suddenly on the ground. Within seconds, we had a dog fight; kids in the middle and I was on the ground stunned with Jade's leash quickly sliding off my hand.

I was told by an onlooker that the black lab approached my other son, Brian. Jade lunged between Brian and this other dog. Jade had never shown any aggression, however, in this new situation, chaotic activity and a new dog approaching his family member; it appears that Jade got defensive. Some friends said that the other dog growled first, but that didn't stop the accusations that came after this was over.

People were throwing things at the fighting dogs, and I heard kids crying, screaming, and shouts to kick the dogs, to which I kept shouting back, not to kick them. As I struggled to get to my feet, the smart person whose house we were in front of, turned on his hose and with a powerful stream of water, startling the dogs long enough so they could be separated. I was shook up, but my adrenalin kicked in as I made sure my children were safe and then retrieved Jade from a neighbor who walked him away from the other dog to the side of the house, a place more safe. This neighbor knew Jade as a friendly dog, and remarked that he wasn't afraid of him, even now. We were all thankful that none of the other dogs out that night joined in on the fight, although you could hear their whines and growls from the distance as their handlers pulled them away from the scene.

My children were scared and crying and Jade was bleeding. With help from friends, we rushed to the emergency animal hospital. Jade had a few scratches to his face and front legs, and kept whining during the examination. The veterinarian said he could be emotionally traumatized by the fight if he thought his "family" was in danger or hurt. He asked us to come into the room to calm Jade. My children had never witnessed a dog fight, much less, their beloved Jade acting so aggressive. With the help of the veterinarian tech, talking about how he thought Jade was acting like his costume and being a good "police" dog, and protecting them, my children began to worry more about Jade and less about the fight. They wanted Jade to know he was still a "good boy" and showed their love for him with hugs, kisses and compliments. This seemed to calm all of them.

While we were at the animal hospital, a police officer came by. Someone had reported the incident and he needed to verify the injuries and my perception of the event. Because of the complaint Jade was taken away by animal control and had to be kept in custody until they could determine what crime may have been committed. It took two days for the police to complete their interviews and determine that it was an accident. No one could account for which dog actually started the fight and no human was injured by the dogs. Several parents were upset at the trauma their children were exposed to and a few were finger pointing at anyone who had a dog out that night. It's caused a little rift in our neighborhood and a couple friendships have gotten cooler.

Jade seemed to be his usual self once he was home again. It took a few months for the replay of the event to fade out of our household and neighborhood conversations. But when Halloween approaches again, the memories resurface. My kids will be in costume again, and we will be going out as a family, however, this time Jade will stay at home.

To Leash or Not to Leash

By Mike Branson

In most cities there are ordinances stating dogs must be leashed anytime they are in public, yet every day I see dogs in stores, on sidewalks, in the street and at the parks (not dog parks); roaming at will, their people often trailing far behind them. Even the best-behaved dogs may occasionally act unpredictably, especially when in unfamiliar territory, frightened or approached by someone they don't trust including hyperactive children. One man I know describes his dog as well-behaved and well-socialized, but once the dog got scared and it bit a child.

I must admit, that it might be cool in some ways if my dog, Blue, was so well trained that he *always* stayed by my side. It would be best if he *always* stopped on command; *always* dropped something he shouldn't have in his mouth; *always* stopped chasing something he shouldn't or *always* came back immediately on the first command. But a roaming cat, a dropped piece of fried chicken, or another dog can supersede my first command and he has graduated from some of the best training classes.

Blue usually accompanies me to one of his favorite places - the pet store. The store has a big sign at the entry that all the dogs must on leash in the store. Last week, a person came in with two large dogs and only one was on leash. The one off leash immediately approached Blue and then growled aggressively. Since Blue was on leash, I could turn him away, but this other dog kept approaching, still growling, and his person seemed clueless. I yelled for her to get her dog and she said, *"Oh, that's ok, he just needs to learn his boundaries."* Huh? Now the store personnel got involved between her dog and Blue and strongly advised her to leash her dog. The woman got upset with the store person that she threw down what she had in her hand, yelled that she would never shop this store again and dragged her still growling dog out by his collar with the other dog tailing behind her being pulled by his leash.

The incident at the pet store was out of the norm seeing a dog off leash, but I see dogs off leash all the time at the family park (not dog park.)

Several days a week I've seen one woman who drives to this park, open her car door and let her little dog loose to chase squirrels. Which he will do non-stop for thirty minutes or more. Sometimes he'll be as far away from her as 100 yards on the other side of the park. She saunters around seemingly keeping an eye on him. One day I overheard someone at the park question her about letting her dog run loose in a park so close to busy traffic. She answered that he likes to chase squirrels and he never goes in the street. Just as the person questioning her said that squirrels run into the street too -

one did! And this dog ran right after it into the street and directly in front of a UPS truck. You could hear dozens of people screaming, but the dog didn't stop. Fortunately the driver of the truck was aware of this area, was driving slow, and was able to stop without hitting the dog. After chasing the squirrel to the other side the street, this little dog didn't miss a beat. He turned around and ran back across the street to where we were in the park. It happened so fast that the UPS truck was still stopped, and he honked his horn, which got the attention of another car that was approaching from the other direction. The only one seemingly unaffected by all the chaos was the little dog who just kept chasing squirrels. It was the gossip at the park for days. We haven't seen this woman and her dog since that day. I hope she is taking him to a fenced dog park to safely do his running.

A friend of mine loves to hike in the nearby mountains with his dogs off leash. Sometimes they stay close to him on the trail, but they have been known to run off into the bushes chasing something they found interesting. He bought one of those GPS systems for his dogs in case they got so far away they didn't come back when he called. These hiking areas have coyotes and mountain lions. A pack of coyotes or a couple of mountain lions can take down most size dogs very quickly. And a GPS isn't going to stop that. As cool as it looks to have his dog run before us on the trail, I'm not comfortable letting my dog loose like that. I've heard too many stories about dogs chasing something into the brush and never returning.

I hear people at the park say it's too hard to control their dog when he's on a leash. Does that mean he's easier to control when they are chasing after him? Maybe they just haven't learned how to leash their dog. Every day I see people jerking their dogs by the collar around their neck. I'm not sure where we got the idea that a dog's neck is as strong as steel, capable of withstanding such force. There are options for dogs that tend to pull, or need correction during an outing, that are designed to be more humane. When Blue and I were first getting used to each other I used an easy-walk, no-pull dog harness on him. The ring to connect the leash is on his chest instead his back. This makes it more difficult for him to pull away. If he does try to pull, the design of this harness guides him back towards me. If we are going to a new park where he might get overly excited or think he's in charge, I'll use this harness.

On regular days, he wears a Martingale collar. Some dogs can back up and pull themselves out of a standard collar. I think this is why some people resort to choke style and spike collars. I just couldn't hurt Blue with something like those. The Martingale collars design makes it impossible for a dog to pull their head out. It's designed, also, not to hurt their neck or throat, or choke the dog. It's a double-loop style collar. One large loop is fitted to Blue's neck size and placed around Blue's neck. His leash is clipped to a ring on a smaller loop. When a dog pulls against his leash, or backs away trying to get his head out, the tension on the leash pulls the small loop taunt. The material from the large loop has now become the extended part of the small loop and this then makes the larger loop tighter. The design of the collar keeps it comfortable, appearing loose, when it's properly sized. If Blue pulls away from me, his collar is pulled to ride around his neck just behind his ears. It's not across his throat so he's not being choked. It's not comfortable for him, so he stops pulling.

He has been trained to respond to the collar being uncomfortable, or the halter preventing him from pulling. Not creating pain or using force to control him. It's less stressful on me to know he's not being hurt.

Like I said, it might seem cool to have my dog off leash, but I'd rather not take the chance of an unexpected event. It's more cool to have him safe and alive.

"A dog is the only thing on earth

that loves you more than you love yourself."

~ Josh Billings

Weather Conditioning

All over the world we have ever changing and some dangerous weather conditions. In the Unites States on the west coast, the earth moves; the desert area temperatures can be severe highs and lows; on the east coast the weather can cause floods, extreme low temperatures and power outages. Around the world weather conditions can have an effect on what your animal companions need from you.

Animals lose most of their body heat from the pads of their feet, their ears, and their respiratory tract. Panting helps them to release body heat in the summer so make sure you have plenty of fresh water available. If you keep a water dish outside for your animal friends, check it often for cleanliness in the summer and make sure it's not frozen in the winter. During hot summer days, the sidewalks can get very hot and they can freeze in the winter. Be aware of how your dog companion is walking on the ground and watch for any discomfort.

Animals left outside will become creative in finding ways to stay warm and cool. Cats will curl up against car engines for warmth. Cats caught in moving engine parts can be seriously hurt or killed. Before you turn your engine on, check beneath the car or make a lot of noise by honking the horn or rapping on the hood. Dogs and cats hide under vehicles, under porches and dumpsters. Be watchful for hiding animals when moving vehicles and trash bins.

Remember to add your cat and dog necessities (ie: sweaters, prescriptions, first aid, food, water, etc.) to your emergency preparedness kits, in your home, at work and in your car. Be prepared. If you're forced to leave your home because you've lost electricity, remember to take your animal companions with you. Keep their leashes and carriers ready and close at hand.

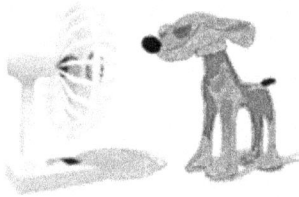

Do You Really Know ?

How hot is it in your car for your cat or dog companion?

It still amazes me how folks will make sure their air conditioner is full blast when they are in the car; and then think nothing of the rising heat inside that same car on their dog when they leave it in the locked car for any period of time.

That "quick" run into the store for one thing can take more time than expected if the store is full and the checkout line is slow, or you remembered one more thing you needed. I can recount several times (without my dog) when I ran into the store, "just for one thing" and ended up spending 30 minutes or longer. Almost everyone has opened a car door and been amazed at the blast of heat which feels much hotter coming from the inside than it is outside. The news channels continue to report the hazards, and then unfortunately also the tragedies of the cats and dogs now ill or dead because people left them in cars ignoring all the warnings.

These excuses, heard most often, don't save the life of a cat or dog left too long in a car in the heat:

"I just ran into the store to buy one thing"

"I parked in the shade"

"I left the windows cracked open"

"I parked in the shade"

Even on a mild day, the temperatures can still rise to deadly levels.

A study from Stanford University School of Medicine[16] shows that even on comparatively cool days, a car's internal temperature will rocket to dangerous temperatures within 60 minutes. They found that, regardless of outside air temperature, the car gained 80% of its final temperature within 30 minutes. And keeping the windows open a crack hardly slowed the rise at all.

After several days of testing, one test indicated that ambient temperature of 66°F outside rose to 84°F inside the car after only 20 minutes. After 30 minutes, it was 93° F inside the car. After 60 minutes, it was over 109° F and still rising.

Their results indicated that:

1.) It doesn't have to be hot outside to be dangerous inside a car.

2.) The temperature spike happens quickly.

3.) Cracking windows doesn't help.

Keep in mind that shade moves. You may be in a shady spot one minute and come back to find your car partially or fully exposed. Even though those windshield sun shades can help keep the car a few degrees cooler, they aren't of much help if the sun is beating down on a side or back window instead. Some car shades have a temperature indicator to let you know it's too hot inside the vehicle.

See it for yourself in your own car and your regular stops - without a cat or dog in the car during your testing. Take an oven thermometer and keep in near where your dog sits in your car. You will be surprised to see how fast the temperature rises.

At least fourteen states (AZ, CA, IL, ME, MD, MN, NV, NH, NJ, NY, ND, SD, VT, and WV) and many municipalities have enacted laws to address the problem of animals left in cars, especially in hot temperatures. Under these laws, police, animal control agents, and others may be authorized to enter the vehicle by whatever means necessary to remove an animal.

If you're out and about on a hot day and see an animal alone in a closed car, you should immediately try to find the car's owner. If you have no luck, or if the owner refuses to act, contact your local police and animal control.

Your dog companions depend on you to keep them safe.

Dog Parks

By Sharone Ray

I live in a small apartment in an area of town where they are very few patches of grass. Dog parks, for me, are the way to give my dog a chance to socialize and play on something other than cement. I've heard pros and cons on dog parks, from dog bites to diseases and fleas, but I believe it has to do with the person's responsibility to find a park that appears clean and watch what and who their dog plays with.

A neighbor takes his dog to a large dog park in the area. This park is one big fenced area for all dogs. With all sizes and temperaments of dogs in one area, his little dog was bit by a much bigger dog. The two dogs were on the other side of the park from where he was sitting, so he doesn't know what sparked the confrontation.

The park I found about a mile from my home has separate areas for little, middle and big sized dogs. One common fence runs between the small and middle sized dogs and some dogs love to fun the length of that fence barking at each other. It doesn't appear to be aggression, only getting their run on. My dog, Henley, is only 12 pounds so we stay in the small dog areas and I keep my eye on him. Last weekend I saw one of the other dogs drooling very heavily. When I asked his guardian what was wrong and he said he didn't know. Without knowing whether this dog was sick, I was concerned and just kept Henley away from him.

When I got home I looked up dog drooling on the internet and read that some degree of drooling is normal in dogs, particularly in breeds with loose lips, like some boxers and bulldogs. This dog at the park was not one of those breeds. Excessive drooling can commonly be triggered by psychological events such as fear, apprehension, and nervous anxiety, as well as anticipation of food treats. This man's dog could have just been excited to be in the park. Drooling also occurs in response to mouth pain caused by periodontal disease, abscessed teeth, and stomatitis, which might have meant this dog needed to visit the vet. Distemper, pseudorabies, and rabies are diseases associated with drooling. A serious disease is what I wanted to avoid. This man didn't know what was wrong with his dog, and frankly, didn't seem concerned. I just kept our distance from them. With dogs and people in a park that I don't know, anything is possible. Not everyone trains their dogs to be well mannered around other dogs either, so I do my best to keep us safe and healthy. Besides, I wouldn't send my child into a play area without being very observant of who she was playing with and what was going on.

Henley and I go to the dog park at least once a week. We go more if the weather is good and I have the energy. He always has the energy. Some of the people sit in chairs under the trees reading books or chatting with each other or on cell phones oblivious to anything around them. I am always within eyesight of Henley so I can see whatever he is doing. When there aren't any other dogs in the park that he wants to play with, we go to a back corner with one of his toys and play toss and fetch. If another dog wants to play with his toy I pick it up. I don't want to take another dog's slobber home with us. Only once, even when no toy was involved, another small dog started to growl and face down Henley; forcing Henley to back up towards a corner. When I saw this I moved in closer the dogs, yelling "hey" at them. Henley didn't take his eyes off the dog aggressing towards him, and the other dog didn't back off.

I always carry Henley's leash as I follow him in the park and a water bottle with a squirt top. When I got close enough I squirted water on the aggressive dog and stomped my feet. That was enough to break his stare and threating stance. I continued to stomp my feet and yell at him until he backed off and ran away. I'm not sure if this would work with bigger dogs, but it was what I was trained to do around little dogs. I hadn't seen Henley get hurt by this other dog, but he looked a little shaken. I reassured him he was safe with me and walked him to another part of the park to play, He seemed alright after that.

A few minutes later a very angry woman approached me asking if I was the one who poured water on her dog. I admitted to squirting him to stop his aggressive approach on my dog. She angrily said that her dog didn't do any such thing. I asked her if she could point out where he was when he got wet. And she said she couldn't. Someone else told her that I made her dog wet. I responded that if she had been watching her dog she would have seen the encounter; and if she was a responsible person, she would have been right there to stop her dog's threatening behavior, I also asked her if she would rather I train my dog to attack so her dog would be bloody instead of just a little damp. She was determined to be angry at me and said she was going to call the cops, which I encouraged her to do. Instead she left the park, but not after telling anyone within earshot what a (expletive) I was. After she left, another woman came to me and said that several people had previous problems with this dog, but no one had ever done anything like that before. She thought it was not only a good idea, but about time. I wasn't pleased to hear this because it meant that some of the people in this park were willing to let dogs get away with bad behavior. I don't want Henley to pick up aggressive behaviors from other dogs. I believe it is my responsibility to watch over him and do my part to help make sure he doesn't cause things like that to happen.

When we leave the park, I always check him for fleas, ticks, scratches and anything caught in his fur. Before he gets into my car I wipe off his fur and paws with a doggie wipes to get a better look. This park has a doggie wash station, just in case Henley gets really dirty, bathrooms for people and lots of safe parking away from the main street. They are closed one day a week so park rangers can clean the area, fill in holes and get rid of weeds and standing water.

I still hear stories about bad things happening at dogs at dog parks, but for me and many apartment tenants, these dog parks are useful. There are so many dogs in my neighborhood, and even more at the local community park on weekends, both on and off leash. I think there is just as much chance of a problem on my sidewalk and at these people parks. I can't change the behavior of other dogs, or their irresponsible humans. Instead, I can keep Henley's vaccinations up to date, teach him good behaviors, watch him closely and check him carefully before we leave for home. We go to the park on non-peak hours, and we leave if we see any aggressive or possibly sick dogs enter. I can keep myself well-informed and trained. Next week Henley and I are going back to training, so I can learn more about how to break up dog fights, and the use of Pepper Spray, just in case. Even after this extra training, I still plan to be just as observant to prevent any problems before they have a chance to start.

"I think dogs are the most amazing creatures;
they give unconditional love.
For me they are the role model for being alive."
-- by Gilda Radner

Car Ride

By Cindy S.

My friend Janie used to always drive with her little Pomeranian, Pookie in the front seat of her car, and usually on her lap. She always told us how cute Pookie looked and how fun it was to have him in her lap. She thought Pookie liked the freedom and since he was so small, only 7 pounds, Pookie didn't get in the way of her driving. She did admit to a traffic ticket for erratic driving one time because Pookie got on the floor near her feet and she kept reaching down to get him back up. She told the cop she was sneezing and that was why she swerved on the road. He must not have bought that story because he gave her an expensive ticket. I was surprised to hear that Pookie didn't get stepped on when she hit the brakes. But even after getting the ticket, she still drove with Pookie on her lap, and sometimes with his head out the driver's side window.

I thought her driving was scary when she was paying more attention to Pookie than the road, so I quit riding with her. If we went anywhere, I drove. If she had Pookie with her in my car, he either stayed in her lap or he didn't come along. Janie thought I was a dog hater, or maybe I hated Pookie. Neither is true.

I got a frantic call from Janie a few months ago. She was on an errand in her car and Pookie was in her lap as usual. She looked away from the road for a second. When she looked back all the cars in front of her had stopped. She had to slam on her brakes really hard to keep from hitting the car in front of her.

In the process Pookie was thrown on across the car and onto the floor with a big thud. When she caught her senses, she could hear Pookie crying and he wouldn't come to her when she called him. He just lay on the floor on the passenger side. She tried to get him up from the floor when she was still seated in the driver's side, but he cried louder when she grabbed for him. She pulled over to the side of the road, got out of the car and went around to the passenger side to get him. He snarled at her when she touched him, so then she knew he was really hurt.

She called me and asked me to go on the internet and find the nearest animal hospital and tell her how to get there. She was crying and scared, so I looked up the nearest place and after giving her directions, I met here there too.

She was so upset, that she ran into the office and screamed for the staff to get her dog from the car. She didn't know how badly he was hurt but his whining was breaking her heart. After a quick inspection, one of the vet techs carefully scooped Pookie off the floor and took him inside. An x-ray showed a fractured leg. I guess Pookie must have hit that floor pretty hard. After Pookie was all fixed up the veterinarian gave Janie a stern talking to. He told her of the many little dogs that get crushed under brake petals, fall out of driver side windows, or get caught in steering wheels and thrown across the car. And it always happens to people that say: *"oh I'm careful that will never happen to my dog."* The vet's scolding left her feeling guilty that she had actually hurt her beloved Pookie with her own silliness.

Janie has three children, so the Vet asked if she would let any of them ride in her lap when she's driving. Fortunately she said she didn't. The Vet reminded her that years ago we used to drive with our small children and babies riding unsecured in the car. It took many accidents and lost lives before some parents understood the dangers of their children not being properly seated in safety seats. Even under protest, laws were enacted to not only prevent serious injuries to the children, but to also make the easier for the driver to have one less distraction. I've seen firsthand with Janie and Pookie, how dangerous it is to drive with a small dog in your lap. The dog is moving around, sometimes trying to get their head and body out the window. Janie was regularly adjusting the open window and rearranging Pookie, to keep her from jumping or falling out. If Pookie moved away from her lap, Janie was looking around the car (instead of the road) to see what Pookie was doing. Sometimes she would be trying to reach Pookie in the back seat, and calling for him to come. It reminded me of when I was a kid and me and my brothers would be fighting in the back seat. My mom would be turning around and reaching for us with that familiar phrase "Don't make me come back there." We always thought it was funny, until mom hit a pole. We never understood why we were blamed for the accident.

Several states are trying to introduce laws to make it illegal to drive with a dog in your lap, but a lot of people are fighting it. I'm not in favor of more laws but when states rely on drivers to have good judgment, some people just don't think how dangerous it is to drive with an animal in their lap. To me, it seems like common sense has gone to the dogs.

This was the wake-up call for Janie. She bought a cute dog booster seat that connects to the car's seat belt and it has a tether for Pookie. The booster seat is raised so Pookie can look or put his head out the side window; but the tether prevents him from getting out of the seat. It has been an adjustment for both of them. After Pookie's leg healed Janie started taking him places again. At first he whined when she put him in the seat and didn't let him roam the car or sit in her lap. I told her to put a picture of Pookie and his leg cast on her dashboard to remind her, just in case she thinks about letting him back in her lap. Warnings from concerned friends and an expensive traffic ticket didn't do it. Unfortunately, Pookie paid the price with an injury before she saw how dangerous it was.

I wish that regardless of how small or well behaved a person thinks their dog is, that they would think more sensibly before driving with their dog in their lap,. With Pookie in his booster seat, Janie drives more calmly and I'm not afraid to ride with her anymore. Overall, we all seem less stressed with this new arrangement.

"If you get to thinkin' you're a person of some influence,

try orderin' somebody else's dog around."

~Cowboy wisdom

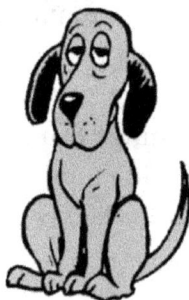

TRAINING

"In order to really enjoy a dog,
one doesn't merely try to train him to be semi-human.
The point of it is to open oneself
to the possibility of becoming partly a dog."
~Edward Hoagland

Mindful Training

In many ways cat and dog lovers will enthusiastically state that their animal companions are better than many people they know.

Although I can't train people to behave a certain way, I can train them how to treat me in the way I state and hold my boundaries. We can learn from cats and dogs how they train each other. Puppies and kittens in the litter teach each other the boundaries of play and space. This is one reason why it is important for them to stay with the litter for a minimum of eight weeks. From mom and their littermates they learn etiquette and socialization. They learn how not to bite too hard, and how to get along with each other. There's also the security of being with their siblings which may ward against some separation anxiety at a later age. A yip or hiss usually signals a boundary. If ignored, a nip or scratch might enforce the message.

Cats and dogs that have been treated abusively do remember who it was that struck them or tortured them. In a future encounter with this person, they may defend themselves, growl to give the message of distrust, and/or attempt to remove themselves from this person's presence whenever possible. Others may become withdrawn and skittish. When animals are raised with abusive techniques it alters their personality.

Just like people, animals can be raised to be mean and distrustful or loving and sweet. It is essential to be mindful and responsible in how we treat those who rely upon us for their safety and guidance.

I have learned helpful information about sharing my home with Tigger and Merlin from a few shows on the television channel Animal Planet. One show, *"My Cat from Hell,"* the cat behaviorist, Jackson Galaxy, always treats the cats with respect and he appears to be able to speak their language. He first listens to the people explain the problem from their perspective and he then offers guidance how to better understand cat behavior in their environment. Not all cat breeds and personalities are the same, so it is not a one-answer-fits-all solution. Sometimes the people need to understand how to make their home more cat friendly; or recognize how their behavior is actually creating or adding to the problem. In one episode a beautiful white cat was saved from being euthanized but he then was thought to be unpredictably mean and a lost cause. The guardians were ready to abandon him. Within a few short weeks, by following Jackson's suggestions on changing how they picked up and held him, plus a few changes in their environment, the cat's loving personality was free to be expressed.

I met Jackson Galaxy at an event at a local shelter. I took the opportunity to ask him about the behavior of one of my cats. One of my cats, Jasper, was peeing in my husband's shoes instead of the litter box. I thought that Jasper just didn't like

195

my husband and was telling him so by taking revenge on his shoes and any clothes he left on the floor. Jackson asked a number of questions about Jasper, such as: when he came into the home, were there any other cats prior to Jasper; how many other cats were in the home with him, and their ages; his overall health and more. Jackson suggested that Jasper was not being revengeful, but was trying to mark his territory. Lancelot and Ariel had come into my home together as kittens. Unfortunately Arial died at 6 months from a shoe string incident. *(See the chapter on Safety.)* Jasper came into my home to be a companion to Lancelot, a few weeks later. It took a couple of days for the hissing to stop, but I thought that the two cats were becoming good friends. Jackson's take was that my home still had the scent of Ariel, and Lancelot was a much larger cat, and followed me around like a shadow. Plus this was a rental home, and it was possible that other animals had lived in it previously. Jasper was looking for places to mark as his, and make this home his as well. Seeing it this way seemed logical, since Jasper was peeing in places that Ariel hadn't been and Lance wasn't interested in. Jackson suggested adding a second litter box in a different room and different cat trees or toys just for Jasper. It had never occurred to me that Jasper might be feeling insecure. It made sense. Just as people may have some questionable behaviors when they are feeling insecure in a relationship or home, so may cats.

One of my other favorite shows, *"It's Me or the Dog,"* uses only positive reinforcement teaching methods. The trainer's techniques require patience to relearn how to train your dog; however, in every episode the end results appear to be lower stress in both people and dogs. I've used some of these positive training techniques with Tigger.

I consider myself very fortunate that he isn't a barking dog. He does not bark at the door, passersby or even other dogs, except when those dogs are on television. It was an unusual kind of bark, kind of a yowl-bark and a lot of bouncing in front of the television. At first I thought it was cute, then it got annoying, because any program with a dog would bring on his nonstop reaction. It began to limit my viewing of some of my favorite shows, including Animal Planet. It was funny when he started barking at cartoon dogs in commercials but now it was really time to do something. Lucky for me, there was an episode on one show that Tigger and *I* both learned from. Tigger loves to sit next to me on the couch, sometimes also chewing on his favorite bone. After watching the show, the next time he started to bark at the dog on television, I used the technique I learned from the show. I said a sharp "ah-ah", picked him up, took him into the next room, set him down, and shut the door with him inside. I went back and sat on the couch for a few seconds. I believe he could hear me walk back to the couch and sit down. Since he's only twelve pounds, picking him up was easy. This might require a ready leash for a larger dog. After the 30 seconds had passed, I got him out of the room and invited him to sit on the couch with me. If he again barked at the television, I repeated the procedure. Yelling at a dog for barking is like barking back at them. They seldom learn that the goal is for them to be quiet.

After only a couple of times, the yowl-barking stopped; and then it was an occasional quiet low growl as he sat next to me on the couch. It's important that I am mindful and anticipate what he is going to see on television. If I'm watching an animal show, I pet him when he is quiet, repeating that he's a good dog. If he would start the low growl, I would say the "ah-ah-ah" and stop petting him. If that didn't work, I would put him on the floor calmly saying "quiet". When he became quiet I would let him back on the couch. If putting him on the floor wasn't enough, then he would be taken out of the room. Sometimes he gets high-value treats when he is on the couch. This works well if a dog is suddenly on the screen and it appears that Tigger is beginning to think about reacting. I let him see the screen and feed him pea-sized treats, repeating calmly, "good boy." I then stop the treats and pet him instead. From the training we received at the shelter, and this show, I learned to vary his rewards so he will respond positively when he gets either treats or attention. So far it's been working. Sometimes the TV will be on and I'll leave the room, only to hear that familiar yowl-bark. I get back to the room as soon as possible and use the removal technique. Whether I am close by or in another room, my desire is for him to feel comfortable with whatever is on the TV screen. This may seem to some to be a lot of work; however, the rewards are a quieter house and the peace to watch the shows I enjoy. A little persistence pays off in a less stressed environment for both of us.

One of my friends growls instead of saying "ah-ah-ah". She said this is what she saw mommy dogs do with their puppies. Her dog listens to the growl and responds by being quiet, or stops whatever behavior he might be doing. I was there one day and felt stressed and frustrated with something I was working on and I growled at my frustration and my computer. Her dog was in the room napping. He got up, looked at me and left the room. I felt he was telling me that he didn't do anything wrong. I quickly found him and gave him love and "good-boys." In afterthought I recognized how he had given me the opportunity to take a break from what I was working on and play with him for a few minutes. When I returned to my project, it seemed to go easier with less stress.

Many of the trainers I've watched or read recommend that if your cat or dog is displaying an extreme behavior, especially if it's new, that you should take them to the veterinarian for a thorough medical check-up. Sometimes a medical condition can be the cause or part of the cause of their disruptive behavior. We don't always act our best when we aren't feeling well.

The training starts the minute you open your home to a new member of the family. When we don't train our cats and dogs, they train us.

Dr. Kim talks about how she trained Shadrach how to sleep in his crate; not to touch certain things; the appropriate place to dig, and more. *"...I trained him from the beginning to not mouth or touch anything in the house; that was easy, since I simply replaced what I didn't want him to touch with something I didn't mind his touching, such as one of his own toys."* (Read her story, earlier in this book: *"Shadrach the Neo Mastiff ... nuthin' but the dog in him!"*)

As a small child my family had a beagle. We didn't train him, but kept him chained to a dog house in the back yard. At the time, we thought it was what we were supposed to do. We thought that only "snooty" people actually let the dogs in their house. Laddie pulled to the extent of his tether to try to play with us kids in the yard. Our backyard was fenced, so there were times we let him off the tether to play. Because he was untrained on how to play appropriately with us and he was so excited to have freedom, we sometimes got hurt by his enthusiasm.

As a teenager, my father had Australian shepherd work dogs and companions. They were indoor/outdoor dogs. They lounged either in the barn or our living room. My father believed that all dogs should be trained, so they were. They listened to his commands alertly and showed a great deal of devotion to him. They watched over our property and protected their domain. They went with us in the pickup truck, slept on the living room floor at our feet and scared the life out of anyone who ventured too far onto our property without first stopping by our front door. Our barn was used occasionally by friends to board their horses. Even as well-known to our dogs as these people might be, the rule was to make your visit known at the house before going to the barn, or find yourself running for safety, as one surprised visitor did. We heard his screams and found him hanging on the side of the hay loft; staring in the faces of snarling dogs who gave every impression those teeth were ready for business. Our dogs never bit anyone; however, you might not believe that if you were the one hanging off the hayloft.

I live on a very busy street, so one of my concerns was Tigger running out and into traffic whenever the front door would be opened. Before adopting him, the shelter taught me and Tigger a few very important commands. This one is "wait". Whenever I open the door, he sits and waits, even if he isn't going out with me. After I walk through the doorway, I tell him "OK", and he then follows me. We've done this so many times that if I forget to say wait, he still sits on the inside until I am through the door and he looks at me for permission to follow. This is not only helpful at home, but anywhere we visit.

It's also important to be mindful of what type of collar or harness to use with your training. This is discussed in the chapter "*Love or Abuse*", and Michael Branson mentions this also in the chapter "*To Leash or Not to Leash.*" I learned recently that a dog in my neighborhood, named Scooter, nearly lost her life under the wheels of a big SUV. Scooter was being taken on her walk when something scared her. When she jumped and pulled backwards away from her person, the collar slipped off over her head. In fear Scooter ran into the street into the path of a large SUV. It was frightening for everyone who witnessed this. The driver did stop in time, and Scooter stopped just short of the vehicle's wheels. The driver was yelling at the dog's person, and the dog's person was yelling back at the driver and calling for Scooter at the same time. Scooter finally responded to her name and the command to come back. She ran back to her person shaking from fear. Up until this point, Scooter had only been trained using one particular type of collar, however, this incident made it apparent that this collar may not be sufficient for her training and her safety. Be mindful to find the style of collar or harness that fits properly. One size does not fit all. It took a few tests before I found the right ones for Tigger.

Be realistic. Most animals need some training, whether by you or a professional, to help them become well-adjusted. Use positive reinforcement instead of yelling and punishment. Be mindful of how you are acting towards them, or expecting them to behave. Most of them don't misbehave because they're bad or trying to displease you. They may be acting out to get your attention, because they're not exercised or stimulated enough; because they're bored or stressed; or because they haven't been trained and they don't know what you want them to do. Effective training takes patience for both of you.

"No Matter how little money
and how few possessions, you own,
having a dog makes you rich."
~ Louis Sabin

Dog Training - For People, Too.

During break time at obedience school, two dogs were talking.

One said to the other...*"The thing I hate about obedience school is you learn ALL this stuff you will never use in the real world."*

I've heard several trainers say that it's not about training the animal - it's about training their person. Dogs don't fail training - it's the handlers who give up.

Just like when we learn a new habit or method, consistency is the key. Our dog companions rely upon us to be consistent with them so that they can learn the instruction or command is important. If, when we learned how to drive, we never heard another instruction or saw a street sign after the initial teaching, our driving would be chaos. We would run through intersections; speed through construction zones; drive on the wrong side of the street and park in the oddest of places (if we actually were able to arrive in one piece). Consistent teaching and reminders help us, and our dog companions, to learn how to live together happily, safely and less stressed.

I see different behaviors every day during my walks with Tigger. From the lady next door who has her dog stop and wait at every corner before crossing the street on her command, to the one across the street who is constantly yelling "*no!*", "*come back here!*", "bad dog," and "*I don't know why he forgot all his training.*" The lady next door and her dog appear to walk leisurely (or run when she's exercising); and they appear to be enjoying their time together. Across the street, she looks haggard and frustrated and her dog cowers each time she yells. They both appear to be experiencing stress.

Enjoy your time together by using consistent training - for both of you. Learn and use methods that work without the use of force, aggression, gadgets, choke chains or fear. Convey your status of leader in a way that is better understood by your dog companion and you will both be less stressed.

Love or Abuse?

Friends and I were looking for dog training shows on television one night. We found a few on different channels. We bounced from one channel to another to see what techniques were being taught. We saw trainers who claimed to use energy to communicate; others using age-old remedies and some showing positive reinforcement training.

On a few shows we were appalled at what we saw. One trainer proclaimed to use invisible energy to communicate with dogs to get them to exhibit the desired behavior. Yet in one session we witnessed a prong choke collar being used. The leash attached was yanked harshly several times raising the dog's feet from the ground. This pulled her back from entering an open door, and was repeated until the dog cowered in submission. In another scene this same dog was hit sharply in the chest with the tips of four tightly positioned straight locked fingers, which again forced the dog to cry out and then become submissive. What we witnessed appeared to be training by fear and aggression, not love. We were uncomfortable watching this show.

We changed channels and watched another show where a dog had suddenly begun to exhibit aggression towards an older dog in the house. I've read reports where this aggressive change from previous friendly behavior could be the result of many different factors, which if the underlying cause is treated, the effect will change. In the show we watched, we didn't see the trainer make any inquiry into what might be the underlying cause, instead the younger dog was treated with harsh handling every time he was near the older dog. It appeared that the idea was to make the younger dog afraid of the older dog through forceful efforts and inducing pain. It was upsetting to watch, so we changed the channel.

These shows claims the training methods are loving. We questioned each other, is what we had watched was really love, or was it fear and intimidation? This appeared to us as being similar to child abuse. The child knowing no other form of love, mistakes abuse for love. However the abuser knows the difference.

In a recent study by University of Pennsylvania[17] researchers studied dog people who use punishment, force, and confrontational or aversive methods to train their dogs. These veterinary researchers found that certain confrontational techniques elicited fear and may lead to owner-directed aggression. The team from the School suggested that primary-care veterinarians advise owners of the risks associated with such training methods and to provide guidance and resources for safe management of behavior problems. I have not yet met a veterinarian that offers such advice. Hopefully there are some that do.

We could accept that some larger and stronger dogs may need a stronger hand to train them, however, more humane, positive and reward based training programs have shown excellent results with all types of behaviors, sizes and breeds of dogs.

On another channel, we watched a show where the trainer was working with a dog who appeared to hate one of the persons in the home. The trainer watched the dog's behavior closely, asked questions about the home; when the problem started; what other changes might have occurred recently and then assessed that the dog was scared and uncomfortable in the environment. This fear was then exhibited as aggression. Seeing the cause of the aggression and not just the aggressive behavior, this trainer used positive reinforced training. After a little time of consistent training, the new dog learned that these people were "safe." afterwards this family was proud to show how the dog happily greeted all members in the home.

Granted, no two dogs or situations are the same. For some people looking for a quick fix, the aggressive move may seem to help. At least in the moment. The research appears to report that a positive approach is more loving and will provide a longer lasting and positive result.

I met a woman at the park who shared with me that she used to use a prong collar on her dog to gain control and get a quick response. She then personally tested the feel of the prong collar on her own skin. It stressed her to think that she was hurting her dog companion; especially when she was impatient and jerked the leash. Even though the dog's skin might be tougher or protected with fur, she switched to a more humane collar and enrolled in more positive leash training. The results, she said, were quicker and they both seem less stressed.

I am cautious to follow advice, whether on television, in a book or class when a disclaimer reads "do not attempt these techniques without consulting a professional". This causes me question of why I'm shown these techniques if they are so dangerous? This type of legal disclaimer is routinely seen on stunt programs showing potentially irresponsible and dangerous actions. This disclaimer is for their protection, not ours. When this disclaimer is on a dog training type show, it gives the impression that it is for the protection of the trainers, not the animals.

When selecting a trainer for your dog, you might consider asking your friends who they used. Before using the same trainer, observe your friends and their dog companions. Are they still following the training, are they enjoying the commands and interaction, or do you witness stress? Just because a trainer seems to have a large client list, it doesn't necessarily mean that their techniques are the best for you to follow; nor does it mean they use techniques that you will find acceptable. A trainer in Colorado made the news when he was arrested and charged with a felony count of aggravated cruelty to animals, for punching and beating his own dog. [18]

Do their words match their actions? If they advertise humane and/or loving training, how do you feel when watching them in action? Would you want this type of training used on you? If you don't want it used on your, then why would you want it used on a animal member of your family?

We are a society that has become numb to the abuse that is inflicted on animals. Every day I witness dogs being yanked by their necks, slapped, held down to force submission and constantly being yelled "no" in their face. People will use harsh treatment on their dogs because it appears to give them a quick result or quick fix. Some people don't know there is another way. Only when enough people challenge questionable treatments will they begin to look for humane training programs. As the safer and more loving treatments become more popular, hopefully they will then become the norm.

"Dogs have given us their absolute all.

We are the center of their universe,

we are the focus of their love and faith and trust.

They serve us in return for scraps.

It is without a doubt the best deal man has ever made."

~ Roger Caras

Rhettung

By Ellen Bishop

My name is German, so is my breed.
I have big ears and ginormous feet.
I sleep on the bed of the boy I protect.
For love and attention, my toys I fetch.
My eyes are brown and filled with glee
Each time he walks in, talking to me.
I wag my tail and clear a nearby table.
I nuzzle my head on his lap as he reads me a fable.
He scratches my ears and kisses my nose.
I paw at his arm and sniff at his toes.
He snuggles me close at the end of the day
No harm will come for I'm in its way

Rhettung came into my life when he was just eighteen months old. He was forty pounds underweight, had the worst habits in the world, and was just a huge puppy. His previous owner had been an elderly gentleman that was no longer able to care for a dog of this size.

After tracking down the family, the daughter informed me that "Buddy" would need a new home and would I see that he found a proper one? I discussed with her my previous Search and Rescue experience, asked if she felt he would need a job, and would she sign him over to me so he would not have to linger in the shelter? She readily agreed. She knew all of his bad habits, including the need to chew everything in sight, have a toy in his mouth always wanting to play, and drinking from the toilet to name a few. I was informed that he had received basic obedience training, but that the training was not continued on a consistent basis. I thought to myself, "Well he has the potential at least, let's see what he's made of."

I brought him home, introduced him to the group, and he was immediately part of the pack. Renegade, my flat coated retriever who was also the alpha and nanny dog, let him know who was boss and that was that. I renamed him Rhettung, which is rescue in German, as he didn't respond to Buddy. He answered to the new name right away.

We began furthering his training, starting with off leash commands then working on to agility. Every chance there was available; we walked with him to the shopping district a few blocks away and introduced him to everyone walking near and to the different sounds and distractions. He never flinched.

As the weeks progressed, I noticed his lack of enthusiasm to find someone hidden for training. My hopes faded; yet I knew this big guy needed a job. After much discussion, we opted to use him as my pet first aid training dummy. I train people how to respond to animal emergencies so this was the perfect opportunity for Rhettung as well. He is the live animal we use in the classes to poke, prod, splint, muzzle, and handle. He also attends community events to bring awareness to emergency responders as an ambassa-dog.

Rhettung is now almost five years old, still romps around the yard like a puppy, loves my son whom he sleeps with every night, and works hard for me. He will always be the biggest baby of the house as he now weighs ninety-two pounds, which is where he should be for a king German Shepherd, but most of all, he is the love that knocks over the baby gate, climbs in your lap like a pup, and kisses your entire face when you least expect it.

"Dogs are not our whole life,
but they make our lives whole."
- Roger Caras

MAKE A DIFFERENCE

A woman and man both arriving in Heaven begged to ask God one question.

They asked, "The world we left had so many animals being euthanized, abandoned and mistreated.

Why didn't you send people to help?"

And God answered, "I did. I sent you."

<u>YOU</u> CAN BE THE DIFFERENCE

If you can - Adopt

If you can - Foster

If you can - Volunteer

If you can - Sponsor

If you can - Donate

If you can - network and spread the word.

There is always something you **CAN** do.

Volunteer

"Volunteering is an act of heroism on a grand scale.

And it matters profoundly.

It does more than help [animals] beat the odds;

it changes the odds."

~ President Bill Clinton

Volunteers can made a huge difference. Animal shelters, like many other nonprofit companies have limited funds and rely upon their volunteers to make up the difference. Just as volunteers can make a difference giving their time and resources to an animal shelter, you can find personal benefits as well. I learned a lot about proper animal care because of my work at the shelter.

In the chapter *"We Saved Each Other's Lives"* I share how I met Tigger because of my volunteer work at a local shelter. Up until my neighbor suggested it, the idea of volunteering at an animal shelter had not even crossed my mind. I had no idea how much it would add to my life.

When I started my volunteer time, I stayed away from the cats. I was still grieving the departure of my beloved Lancelot. Until one day when they received a couple of litters of kittens, all ill and very much in need of help. Because of their apparent health conditions some places may have taken the short route and euthanized these little beings. Not this place. Every day these kittens received what they needed in order to help them build their immune systems and regain their health.

During the weekdays there are fewer volunteers, which is when I am usually there. I was asked to assist with the kittens. Since I was avoiding the adult cats, the kittens seemed safe. There were so many of them. They were all so cute. As they got healthy, they became very lively and rambunctious. It took at least two people at the same time to enter the cat house to block and catch the kittens as they raced to escape through any open door.

Anytime someone entered their room it was also an instant ankle attack as they ran over in mass seeking affection. Great care had to be taken not to let any of them escape to the main room; however, occasionally one or two would shoot through our legs so fast you only saw a blur. Attempting to corral kittens was worthy of America's Funniest Videos. We would scramble to catch the fuzzy bullets and laughing the entire time at ourselves and the kittens. You could not be stressed at so much activity and cuteness.

I met other volunteers and heard how being a volunteer had enriched their lives. Stacy wasn't allowed to have any animals in her apartment, so she spent every evening after work at the shelter getting her cat fix. Marcia devoted her time to the dogs. She attended every dog training class the shelter offered, learned how to properly walk a dog and how to earn their trust. She was between jobs and it gave her the motivation to expand her job search to animal related companies. Tom and Nancy met as volunteers and are now happily married for over five years. Jonathan's wife has allergies to animals, so he spends his free time caring for and playing with the dogs. He brings a change of clothes so when he goes home he doesn't carry in anything that would be a problem for his wife. Trish got over her shyness when she was called upon to assist with the shelter tours. Bonnie was getting over a difficult divorce and had become a recluse. Volunteering on adoption days helped her to become social again and meet new friends.

There are shelters in every city. Each one has different needs and requests. Check to see how you can help them. You may enjoy how it changes your life.

Making a Difference

By Lynda Fishman

Air Canada flight 621 crashed on July 5, 1970, killing all 109 passengers and crew members. In that plane crash, I lost my mother and two younger sisters. At 13 years of age, I was faced with the ominous responsibility of a father in a complete state of despair, a house to take care of, and what felt like hundreds of well-meaning relatives and friends telling us exactly what to do and how to proceed with our shattered lives. My life completely collapsed around me, and hope seemed out of reach, but I took baby steps. I refused to give up. I never let go of my faith in the future. Somehow I intuitively knew that despite the pain, I could make some good choices, and create my own journey.

I came from a home that valued family, charity, gratitude, faith and integrity. As kids, we watched as our parents lived purposeful lives where they reached out to others, helping, guiding, and comforting. My parents were always involved in charity events and volunteer work. We didn't have much money, but our home and our lives felt rich and abundant. We were a family of action, committed to learning, growing and making a difference. I have learned through the years that one of the most effective ways of dealing with a difficult situation is to be busy or distracted. Too much time to "think" can be very dangerous. The greatest gift we can give to ourselves is a project or activity that keeps us busy and is extremely pleasurable at the same time.

A few months ago, someone left a box of young kittens on the side of the road near my summer day camp, Adventure Valley. Since there are no coincidences in life, I believe it was meant to be that someone just happened to walk by and heard the kittens crying in the box. Next thing I knew, I was at the veterinarian with three young, healthy and adorable kittens. I saw this as a gift from the Universe – an opportunity to make a difference. It is remarkable how animals have such a natural ability to show gratitude and appreciation.

The veterinarian told me that there is a desperate need for foster homes for kittens, and that because of the shortage of foster homes, healthy kittens are being euthanized every day. We immediately transformed my daughter's bedroom and adjacent washroom into a kitten nursery – litter box, food and water bowls, a cozy pet bed and plenty of toys. The kittens required a lot of time and attention, but they were an absolute joy. Within a few weeks they were chubby and old enough to be adopted. We found wonderful homes for them and have heard from the adoptive families that they are cherished pets.

We have since then become an official kitten rescue home and received a new litter of four very young kittens who were left in a box outside of a well-known pet store. We bottle fed and litter trained these tiny kittens; and have watched them grow into absolutely adorable and affectionate little pets. They love playing together and zooming around chasing each other. They are in great health, fully litter box trained, playful, cuddly, entertaining and very social. They love lots of attention! It is a delight to be busy looking after these kittens and I look forward to finding wonderful homes for them.

When you first look at a litter of tiny kittens, the work and time needed for their care can seem overwhelming. That's where my sense of determination and the desire to take on a challenge jumps in! The idea of helping, doing something worthwhile, and succeeding - fuels me to JUST DO IT!

Nothing builds self-esteem, self-confidence and the feeling of empowerment like a meaningful challenge followed by accomplishment. Realizing that you have the desire and ability to care for tiny, dependent little kittens, and that because of your tender love and care, they can be healthy, content and playful, is incredibly rewarding. When you rescue kittens, you're doing something important. You are giving these animals a second chance. You're keeping them alive. They depend on you – and they will love and appreciate you unconditionally.

To learn about Lynda Fishman, visit the "About the Authors" section in the back of this book.

Foster Parents

By Ellen Bishop

They open their lives, their homes and their hearts
So forgotten animals can be given a start
They love and nuzzle and treat them with care
So someday a real home they can finally share
Up half the night with chances so slim
Never a thought to the light growing dim
They fight and they battle for what is right
For some poor soul left out in the night
The hours are long, the work with despair
Yet they trudge on, ever hopeful out there
To help just one more creature in life
To learn about love and leave behind strife.

Foster parents open an entirely new option for a shelter or rescue. They open their hearts, homes, and wallets for a strange animal to come into care and be saved from certain death. They take on the ones that staff feel need help. The animals' ages range from days old to extremely senior.

A foster family dedicates their time to ensuring that the creature learns compassion and obedience that will enable it to move to a permanent family prepared to be a pet. They take the animal to veterinarian appointments, classes, out into the general population for socialization, and for exercise. In many cases, the family chooses to pay for the expense of a foster animal from their own pocket to save the shelter resources to care for other animals that are not able to find a foster or permanent home.

Most animals that come into foster care require not only medical attention but also patience. Their behavior may be erratic, their trust for humans wary. They have not been shown the love that teaches them security and therefore, they act as they would if left in the wild on their own. They tend to chew, mark their territory in different ways, and not have the manners of those who that have known a loving hand from infancy. Yet, with the care and guidance provided by a family, they begin to become the beloved pet a permanent home will care for through the days of life.

See the Authors section at the back of the book to learn more about Ellen Bishop

Rescues

By Ellen Bishop

We take your tired, neglected, unwanted, and abused
To show them love, attention, care, and hope.
We have them spayed or neutered and do what we can
For their health and emotional healing to begin.
We struggle knowing there are many and we can
*   only help few*
Our time and money is worth more than gold to them.
Our emotions and lives revolve around the animals
*   in our care.*
We give all we have and more each day as it comes
We cling to the hope that someday we will no longer be needed
Knowing that the future is uncertain for most.
We search for a home to accept these outcasts of society
And struggle with knowing all we do will never be enough.
We strive to make a difference and change perceptions
Giving everything we have to let one more live.

Rescues, in my opinion, are the greatest givers when it comes
to animal care outside of a shelter. They sacrifice literally

everything they have at their disposal to help care for the animals our society casts aside. They operate on a budget of donations and their own privately earned funds to help the animals we have abandoned and neglected. They step in when there is little or no hope for an animal in a shelter situation. They take the worst of those and gently see that they are rehabilitated to become caring pets, successful therapy animals, and contribute to the society that had forsaken them.

A rescue staff is comprised of volunteers on a mission to change the world one animal at a time. They spend tireless hours focused on the business at hand. They are caring for those already under them, phoning shelters, setting up transportation, attending vets' appointments, visiting potential homes, and looking for funding options. Most of these duties fall in addition to a regular paying position to support the volunteer work involved with a rescue. A rescue alone or as a community is a formidable opponent. They are often the loudest voice in the court and media crying for a change in the view of treatment. They are also the ones working hard behind the scenes to ensure that the changes are enforced. They have the right to be heard because they are the organization that handles the detail day after day, night after night.

See the Authors section at the back of the book to learn more about Ellen Bishop

Puppy Sighs

Original Author unauthenticated

This is one of the neatest stories, I've received it in an email. It touches my heart every time I read it. You will know precisely what this little girl is talking about at the end.

****

"Danielle keeps repeating it over and over again. We've been back to this animal shelter at least five times. It has been weeks now since we started all of this," the mother told the volunteer.

"What is it she keeps asking for? "the volunteer asked.

"Puppy size!", replied the mother

"Well, we have plenty of puppies at this shelter, if that's what she's looking for. "

"I know...we have seen most of them," the mom said in frustration.

Just then Danielle came walking into the room with another volunteer, having just visited the rooms with the available dogs. The two women looked at each other, shook their heads and laughed.

"You never know when we will get more dogs. Unfortunately, there's always a supply," the volunteer said.

Danielle took her mother by the hand and headed to the door. *"Don't worry, I'll find one when we come back this weekend,"* she said.

Over the next few days both mom and dad had long conversations with her. *"We don't want to hear anything more about puppy size either,"* Mom added.

Sure enough, they were the first ones in the shelter on Saturday morning. By now Danielle knew her way around, so she ran right for the section that housed the smaller dogs.

Tired of the routine her mom sat in the small waiting room at the end of the first row of cages. There was an observation window so you could see the animals during times when visitors weren't permitted.

Danielle walked slowly from cage to cage, kneeling periodically to take a closer look. One by one the dogs were brought out and she held each one. One by one she said, *"Sorry, you're not the one."*

It was the last cage on this last day in search of the perfect pup. The volunteer opened the cage door and Danielle carefully picked up the dog and held it closely. This time she took a little longer.

"Mom, that's it! I found the right puppy! He's the one! I know it!" she screamed with joy. *"It's the puppy size!"*

"But it's the same size as all the other puppies you held over the last few weeks," Mom said.

*"No not size... the **sighs**! When I held him in my arms, he sighed,"* she said.

"Don't you remember? When I asked you one day what love is, you told me love depends on the sighs of your heart. The more you love, the bigger the sighs!"

The two women looked at each other for a moment. Mom didn't know whether to laugh or cry. As she stooped down to hug the child, she did a little of both.

"Mom, every time you hold me, I sigh. When you and Daddy come home from work and hug each other, you both sigh. I knew I would find the right puppy if it sighed when I held it in my arms," she said. Then holding the puppy up close to her face she continued, *"Mom, he loves me. I heard the sighs of his heart!"*

Close your eyes for a moment and think about the love that makes you sigh.

"Life is not measured by the breaths we take, but by the moments that take our breath away."

Always a supply ... It is estimated that animal shelters care for 6-8 million dogs and cats every year in the United States, of whom approximately 3-4 million are euthanized. Visit a shelter to find one that sighs in your arms.

"It is one of the most beautiful compensations of life, that no person can sincerely try to help another without helping themself."
~ Ralph Waldo Emerson

SAYING GOODBYE

"Many who have spent a lifetime in it can tell us less of love than the child that lost a dog yesterday."

~ Thornton Wilder

"A Dog's Purpose"

(lesson from a 6 year old)

This was shared with me this morning from a friend. My dog companion, Tigger, thought I should share it with you.

"Being a veterinarian, I had been called to examine a ten year old Irish Wolfhound named Belker. The dog's people, Ron, his wife Lisa, and their little boy Shane were all very attached to Belker and they were hoping for a miracle.

I examined Belker and found he was dying of cancer. I told the family we couldn't do anything for Belker, and offered to perform the euthanasia procedure for the old dog in their home.

As we made arrangements, Ron and Lisa told me they thought it would be good for six year old Shane to observe the procedure. They felt as though Shane might learn something from the experience.

The next day, I felt the familiar catch in my throat as Belker's family surrounded him. Shane seemed so calm, petting the old dog for the last time, that I wondered if he understood what was going on. Within a few minutes, Belker slipped peacefully away.

The little boy seemed to accept Belker's transition without any difficulty or confusion. We sat together for a while after Belker's death, wondering aloud about the sad fact that most animal lives are shorter than people lives.

Shane, who had been listening quietly, piped up, "I know why!"

Startled, we all turned to him. What came out of his mouth next stunned me. I'd never heard a more comforting explanation. It has changed the way I try and live.

He said, "*People are born so that they can learn how to live a good life -- like loving everybody all the time and being nice, right?*"

The six year old continued, "*Well, dogs already know how to do that, so they don't have to stay as long.*"

Miracle's Last Miracle

By Dr. Joy Vanderbeck

My wonderful and faithful dog Miracle recently made her transition.

Miracle had lost her hearing several months previous. I asked myself if it bothered her that she couldn't hear any longer Tisha, my very in tune daughter in love, had some time alone with Miracle. I knew that Tisha sensed that Miracle wouldn't be with us much longer, but in her wisdom, she didn't mention it to me until much later.

What I observed during the months that followed answered my question. I watched her lose her zest for life. I sensed that she felt as though her purpose as a protector had diminished. I watched as she grew tired earlier and earlier during our walks. Then, Miracle was given a terminal diagnosis.

I know that we are Spirit and beyond diagnoses and prognoses. I have known people who have made a decision to live after receiving a "terminal" diagnosis. Multiple times I have witnessed the correlation between a person's or a pet's will to live and the state of their health.

I also believe in the eternity of all life.

I sat with Miracle on the floor and told her that if she wanted to live, she was going to have to live up to her name and pull off a Miracle. She continued to dwindle and lose her hold on life. I sensed that she was torn between staying with me and coming back and getting to be a puppy again.

I was determined to let her go if that was what she wanted to do. Many times I held her and thanked her for all that she had brought to me and to my clients who loved her dearly. I told her over and over that it was okay to go, and that while I would grieve and miss her, I was willing to let her go. Something that my son Sunny said really helped me with this readiness. Sunny asked me if I could let her go so that some other "old soul dog" could come and share some good times with me. Sunny, too, knew she would be leaving. Sunny commented that at a time like this, my spiritual beliefs would be challenged. He was correct.

The last month of her life became very stressful for me because her appetite changed and what she would eat varied from day to day. For a mom type person, not being able to get my dog to eat was upsetting. I knew what it meant. She was preparing to leave.

I was in a lot of fear that it would be her time to go, and would need help doing so, and I wouldn't get it. While I teach and totally know that saying "I don't know" closes the door to the answer, I kept saying "What if I don't know?" It was a huge issue for me accompanied by many tears. I wanted to do it right for her; I wanted to be spiritually in tune. But I didn't feel in tune. I didn't trust myself with this important decision. I wanted to do it right by my precious Miracle.

Saturday night before she transitioned, she had become so weak that she fell on my kitchen floor and couldn't get up. She lay there with legs spread, whimpering, and unable to get herself up. The whimpering told me that she needed help. I held her and asked her to please go without my having to make the call to euthanize her. I lay blankets all over the hardwood floors to help her have some traction so it wouldn't happen again.

I called the vet the following Monday morning. Miracle was better that day and I told the vet, "Today is not the day." I emailed my Native American friend Cherri and asked her if she could be with Miracle at noon on Wednesday, two days later. She agreed. How did I know that?? I suspect that, while I kept being afraid that I wouldn't know, I kept affirming that I WOULD know. I affirmed that I would know what was best. I affirmed that I would know when it was time.

Still, I kept being in fear and angst about "What if I don't know."

On Tuesday evening, Miracle let herself outside and didn't have the strength to get back inside. I let her in and she was so cold, and didn't warm up as she normally would. I covered her with heavy towels. I knew Miracle's hold on life was very thin, and that her circulation was shutting down.

234

The greatest blessing she gave me that night was creating space for me to hold her and say my farewell. I realized that all through that time, I had told her it was okay to go but I hadn't told her goodbye. I did so that night and it felt awful. It felt horrible. I hate goodbyes. Goodbyes have been a huge trauma for me in my life and here it was again. It dawned on me that it wasn't really goodbye, because at some time we will see each other again in this life or another. I changed it to "See you later" and I felt peace.

I told her to be sure and pick a family next time who would be good to her and love her as much as I did.

The next morning, I awakened, and heard the words of my guidance, "It's time." Then I heard her crying at the back door to come in. Again, she was too weak to come in on her own. I listened to my guidance, and made arrangements for the vet, Cherri, and my son Christian to be here.

Miracle came in to greet and share love with my clients all that morning. The clients were all so in tune that they knew she was leaving though I said nothing. Miracle's last act of service was sharing love with a client who had been horribly abused in his childhood who is struggling to get his heart back. I took pictures. Miracle only had a few minutes left on this earth and one more time, she was helping someone get their heart back.

Miracle's passing was peaceful and she was surrounded with so much love, prayers and Native American blessings.

That afternoon, I was in session with clients and I felt her spirit so strongly. There will always be a connection of love.

I am so thankful that she helped me get yet another part of my heart back. It really IS okay to say goodbye because all goodbyes are really "see you later." And perhaps, since Miracle had been an abandoned dog, we all, through loving her, helped Miracle get her heart back as well.

Thank you Miracle!! Thank you!!

See "About the Authors" section to learn more about Dr. Joy Vanderbeck

"You think dogs will not be in heaven? I tell you, they will be there long before any of us."

~ Robert Louis Stevenson

Love and Saying Goodbye

By Tammy Lawrence-Cymbalisty

When my roommate came home with a rescue cat for me I was thrilled. Unable to come up with a name for her we called her P.C. – short for President's Choice the "no name brand" cat. Not very original but it seemed to fit.

We soon realized it was impossible to keep this cat indoors. There were four of us sharing the home; some more aware keeping the four legged addition inside than others. P.C. was constantly outside. So it was no surprise to us when we discovered she was pregnant. She ended up having four kittens; a stillborn, one female and two males.

Shortly after they were born we soon realized there was something wrong. The kittens were not using their back legs. The vet told us to put the kittens down. He said there was no way they would survive.

It turned out that P. C. had distemper, a viral infection affecting cats. "Of affected kittens that are two months or less of age, 95% die regardless of treatment." (Source: Wikipedia.org). We decided we'd take them home and decide later. If truth be told there was no way we even considered it! If they were meant to live, they would. And live they did!

It wasn't long before they learned to use their back legs. Suddenly we had a household full of mischief. Curtains were not safe, nor shoes, nor countertops...I think you get the point. At ten weeks we adopted out the female and kept the two males; Axel and Chimo.

Years passed. The boys saw me through thick and thin. They sat with me through tears of joy and of sorrow. For many years they were my best friends. Thankfully cats can't tell secrets!

Sixteen years later Axel took himself off of his food. It was a bad sign. After many tests they discovered he had feline leukemia. When I explained his medical history to the veterinarian, she said he could very well have had it his whole life. She said, "Many cats can live for years without exhibiting symptoms."

We were heartbroken. I wasn't sure how I was going to go on without my four-legged best friend. However, we also knew there was nothing we could do about it.

The day came for us to put Axel down. I sat with him holding his paw whispering and sobbing the whole while.

It was so peaceful. When they say you put the animal to 'sleep' it really is that way. He laid down his little head and floated away.

I was about to leave, to go home and cuddle Chimo like never before when the veterinarian tech stopped me.

"You have a cat at home still right?" she asked.

"Yes, his litter-mate" I responded through red swollen eyes. "They haven't been apart once in 16 years."

"How strong do you feel?" She asked.

I looked at her thinking, "How strong do you think I feel?", yet said nothing.

She explained that if I felt strong enough I should take Axel home with me and show Chimo.

Cats need closure also.

Bringing Axel's body home was the last thing I wanted to do. You see it was still winter here in Ontario so we couldn't bury him outdoors. I decided to have him cremated. Yet at that point the only thing that mattered was Chimo. I had to get out of my own way.

The veterinarian tech put Axel in a box covered with the towel from home he had come with. We tucked him safely into the car. I'm not even sure how I drove home that day, but I do know it wasn't about me at all. At that point I didn't matter.

I brought Axel into the house, set the box down on the floor and called for Chimo. When he rounded the corner my stomach sank and tears began to fly. Chimo walked over to him, sniffed just once then walked the other way.

I must have looked like a crazy woman. I went and picked up Chimo and brought him back to the box.

"He's gone buddy," I told him. Chimo walked away as if to say, "Yeah, I see that."

Chimo never once looked for Axel. He never called for his brother either. He got it. And although he grieved in his own way we got closer than we'd ever been.

It was the best advice I had ever received. I encourage you, if you have multiple pets and one passes be sure to show it to the others in your home. They too need closure.

I was so sad to see Axel leave; yet somewhere inside I was equally happy. If we had listened to the veterinarian so many years earlier we would have not had a wonder-filled sixteen years with such a fantastic little soul.

Chimo lived until he was 19 years old and passed of old age. It was equally hard to see him leave.

Last year we started the journey again this time with two eight week old girls from the shelter; Sophie and Bella. They add such joy (oh and mischief...did I mention mischief? I've forgotten how busy kittens can be!)

See "About the Authors" section to learn more about Tammy Lawrence-Cymbalisty.

"With the qualities of cleanliness, affection, patience,

dignity, and courage that cats have,

how many of us,

I ask you,

would be capable of becoming cats?"

~ Fernand Mery

Finding Grace

By Dr. Joy Vanderbeck

My old dog Miracle's ashes were spread, blowing in freedom to the four winds. I was now ready for a new dog. Cherri had spoken the word for my next dog a few minutes after Miracle passed. I heard her words, but my heart wasn't into it and I wasn't ready.

Almost a month had passed since Miracle's departure. As the days went on, I had been feeling the hole in my heart and in the heart of my clients that Miracle's passing had left more and more. My clients adored her, and wept for her passing. I went on Petfinders.com. I registered with Adoptapet.com. I spent hours cruising through the pictures of hundreds of dogs needing homes. I stared at the screen, knowing that my perfect dog was out there somewhere and I just wasn't finding her. The more I looked the more ready I felt to accept a new dog into my heart and into my space. I felt a connection with a dog through the ethers. I could feel her sweet heart. I sensed that her owners couldn't keep her. I saw a red collar around her neck. I knew that the dog that was to be "my" dog was a female Lab. I just couldn't seem to find her! One night,

I was going through the countless pictures and descriptions and I felt a profound sense of longing. It felt as though I was trying to make something happen. I was coming from lack. I was efforting ....and I KNOW better. I felt like a love addict longing and desperate for love.

I knew that Miracle was in Spirit, yet I had the box of ashes I needed to do something with. I have a client whose husband had passed last summer. She had spread the husband's ashes and felt such freedom from doing so. My client challenged me as to why I hadn't done something with Miracle's ashes. On Sunday I realized that my client was coming in the next day, and there was no way I was going to admit to her that I hadn't dealt with those ashes. So spread them I did. I was surprised that the ritual was as heartfelt as it was. I experienced a "final honoring" of my beloved pet.

On Monday night, I called Cherri. Cherri is Native American and is very in tune with animals. I told Cherri that I was now ready for my dog. I spoke my word that the dog that was perfect for me in every way would find her way to me or I to her. I spoke my word with authority and clarity.

The very next day, Cherri received an email from a friend. The friend's email had a list with pictures of 10 dogs needing homes. Cherri usually deletes these, but this time, she decided to send me the email. Cherri's note said, "Be sure and check out #9." Dog #9 was a black male Lab in Sulphur Springs Texas, and was being housed at the Sulphur Springs Animal Control Shelter. Even though I wanted a yellow female Lab, I didn't want to be hard headed, and I wanted to be open to the possibilities of my good, perhaps coming to me in ways that I could not see. I called and left a message. The following day I received a call from a woman, Cindy, who said that Denise at the shelter had called her and related to her that I was looking for a yellow female Lab. Cindy said that she had a young female Lab that she could no longer keep. As Cindy told me the story about her dog, I knew that she was the dog I had been looking for. I was so excited I could hardly stand it. Then I thought, "When will I ever have time to make the 2 hour drive to Sulphur Springs to get her?" As I was finishing my thought, Cindy said, "We will be happy to bring her to you." Wow. How easy was all that??

I had been sitting there for countless hours ...... efforting ...... and all I had to do was speak my word with 100% conviction, and my dog was there with me in the blink of an eye. I named her Grace. She is wonderful!

See "About the Authors" section to learn more about Dr. Joy Vanderbeck

ANIMAL PROTECTION

"The greatness of a nation and its moral progress can be judged by the way its animals are treated."
~ Mahatma Gandhi

First Registry for Animal Abusers

The Animal Legal Defense Fund (ALDF) is making an effort aimed at creating public registries in each state of anyone convicted of felony animal abuse. This could include violence (torture, mutilation, intentional killings, etc.), sexual abuse, and animal fighting as well as neglect (such as hoarding). The ALDF website: http://ExposeAnimalAbusers.org provides extensive information about registry bills, and links for concerned citizens to contact their own legislators in support of abuser registries. Such registries will help protect animals, animal guardians and communities by preventing repeat offenses from anyone with an established history of abusing animals.

Arizona legislatures hope to create an animal abuse registry to aid those selling pets with HB 2310. This bill failed in its initial appearance before a House committee, but attempts are being made to change some of the language so it could still become law. A task force focused on preventing animal cruelty has found what it says are shortcomings in state animal-cruelty laws that have enabled some suspects to avoid prosecution. They are working to define what constitutes cruel confinement, abandonment, neglect and shelter for an animal.[19, 20]

Laws relating to animals can vary widely from state to state. To know the laws in your state, visit this website: http://www.aspca.org/Fight-Animal-Cruelty/Advocacy-Center/state-animal-cruelty-laws.aspx

Some states have very lenient laws; others it's a misdemeanor; and in some states animal cruelty is a Class 1 felony. Check out the laws in your state. If the laws in your state need more support to become updated to stronger enforcement and/or punishment - contact your local elected officials. Don't just call or write once. Call and write often. Get a group to write. Get on the agenda and attend political meetings. By your consistent voice and involvement, show that cats and dogs deserve to be treated with loving care.

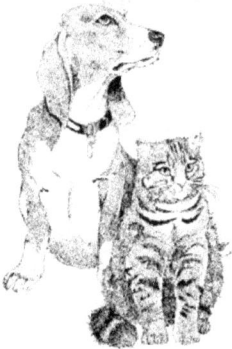

Animal History Disclosure

A new law in Illinois requires pet stores, animal shelters and animal control agencies to disclose pertinent information about an animal.[21]

The following information must be posted on or near an animal's cage: retail price, including additional charges; breed, age, date of birth, sex and color of the dog or cat; details of vaccinations and health history; the name, address and identification number of the breeder and details of any inoculation or medical treatment received while at the facility. Even though pet stores are required to disclose this information if it is requested by the consumer some pet stores do not share it until after the sale is final.

This information will not guarantee a completely healthy long term animal/person relationship; however, it may help some consumers with their decision, and protect them from unknowingly purchasing a puppy mill dog. For those that adopt from shelters and rescues, the medical history is usually limited. The connection and love for the animal carries more weight than the need for medical history.

Disclosure of an animal's age and health is required throughout the United States. Certain states, such as Illinois, Ohio, Maine[22] and California have additional requirements.

California: Retailers must provide each pet buyer with a written form documenting the animal's medical history; retailers also must post the animal's state (or nation) or origin on each cage or display container. When you read Dina's Story *"How Much Is That Doggie in the Window,"* you will see how the information she received may not have been accurate, and she and Georgio paid a hefty price. In Los Angeles there is also a city wide ban on stores to prevent them from sell commercially bred cats and dogs.[23]

Ohio: Any seller (retailer or otherwise) must inform the prospective buyer if the animal has ever attacked or attempted to attack an individual; if so, the seller must describe the event in detail (this information is filed with the local board of health and provided to the buyer- ONLY if it was provided to them.)

In Idaho a felony animal cruelty bill awaits the Governor's signature.

Connecticut is working on a bill that prohibits pet shops from selling dogs and cats obtained from substandard domestic animal mills. One question here is the definition of "substandard domestic animal mills."[24]

It's sad that we need legislation to force people to treat animals with respect and love. We need more states to take a stand against Puppy Mills; to protect animals from abuse and unsuspecting people from purchasing these animals. Contact the animal welfare organizations and elected officials in your area and demand change.

" How we behave toward cats here below determines our status in heaven."
~ Robert A. Heinlein

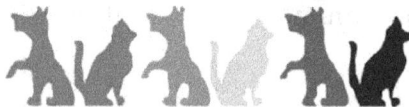

RESOURCES

"If having a soul means being able to feel love
and loyalty and gratitude,
then animals are better off than a lot of humans."
~ James Herriot

How to Adopt your Perfect Cat or Dog Companion

As I said in the introduction, before adopting your (next) cat or dog, ask yourself if you are committed to be in it for the long haul. Many cats and dogs can live fifteen years or more. These days some relationships including careers and marriages don't last that long. During the lifetime of your animal companion you may experience many life changes, such as moving to a new home, changing or losing your job, relationship transitions and other life events. In addition you and/or your animal companion may have medical problems or other adjustments. Are you willing to commit to your companion, no matter what? If it doesn't work out or you change your mind, there is no such thing as kitty annulment or doggie divorce and you both move on to new partners. One of you may not survive the breakup. Our shelters and rescues are bursting at their seams. Thousands of cats and dogs are euthanized every week at animal shelters across the country because of the over population and the lack of funds to care for these discarded friends. These animal companions will love you for their lifetime, and they hope you will return the same love.

When you know you have the commitment, open your heart to the idea that maybe the "type" of cat or dog you think you want, may not be the best one for you and your home, or the one that needs you the most..

I never saw myself as having a small dog in my home. After growing up with large shepherds and working dogs, I always assumed (if I ever got over my fear) it would be a large dog in my home. On the other hand, I always thought those little fluffy dogs were cute (shih-Tzu, Bijan, etc.) but I also saw how much grooming is required. Some people wrongfully think that all cats are aloof or that all dogs are high maintenance. All cats and dogs have different needs and personalities, just like people.

Be mindful of your life, your home and your expectations before choosing your cat or dog companion.

Do your research. If you've never lived with a cat or dog companion consider volunteering for a few months at your local shelter or rescue organization. Get to know how you feel with different breeds, sizes and personalities.

Dogs
Some dogs need room to run, so a person with an active lifestyle might be the best fit.
Some need to dig, so a safe yard might be a solution.

Some are lap dogs or couch potatoes, which might be a perfect companion to an elderly person or someone that is home a lot.

Some are barkers, so understanding this might eliminate stress.

Some dogs are shy and need a patient guardian that will shower them with love and help them to re-learn trust.

Some dogs are very active and want to play all the time. They need a guardian who is active and will take the time to play with them.

Working or hunting breed dogs need an active guardian that can train with them and keep them occupied
Cats:

Some cats need to climb, so having the room to provide them safe climbing spaces would be helpful.

Some need many places to hide, and being aware of the hiding places in your home and making sure these areas are clean and safe will be less stressful for both of you.

Some cats want to be on your lap or in your bed, or where ever you are. These cats are perfect for the person who wants a warm ball of love next to them all the time.

Some cats are more inquisitive and need a home that has safe areas to explore and where dangerous items and products have been removed.

Some cats and dogs need to be the only animal in the home.

Instead of attempting to force a cat or dog to be what you want it to be, accept the best one for your home, your personality, your time and your abilities.

Make your choice with an open heart and an open mind.

When NOT to Adopt a Cat or Dog

There are times that adopting an animal companion is NOT a good idea.

Some of these reasons include:

You've never had a cat or dog in your home and you are going to "try it out." Cats and dogs are not like an outfit you can return if you don't like it later or after the party. A commitment to an animal companion is for a lifetime; Your lifetimes together or the ending of one when you discard them.

You feel sorry for them. Cats and dogs can tell the difference between pity and love. Many times pity becomes a chore and the pity turns to resentment. Love will overcome any bumps in the journey you take together.

On a whim, because you are bored with your life, or think an animal companion will fix everything. Cats and dogs bring a heart full of love, and they can give you another reason to get out of bed, take a walk and get involved. However, they cannot "fix" your life, or relationship. If your life is filled with turmoil, find the appropriate support you need first. Make sure your heart and home are ready for the commitment to the animals, their needs and the changes that will happen in your life together.

When you want to surprise someone at the holidays or their birthday. The adorable furry friend may get oooh's and aaah's when they jump from the box, or you lead them into the room, however, unless you are willing to accept the responsibility of the animal if something changes for the person you are giving them to - then don't do it. Giving one as a gift to a friend can end badly for the animal. When someone is moved to have an animal companion, they take the steps for themselves. Many parents have bought a child a dog and after a few weeks, the child turns their attention to something else and the adult now has all the responsibility of care and training. If you are considering adopting a cat or dog for your child make it a family event. Take the time together to research and then choose the best one for the family.

When you cannot afford it. If you are struggling to make ends meet, then how will you feed your animal companion? Some shelters offer assistance with food and medical care when you adopt from them, however, most of them are counting on donations to help them with the animals who they are saving.

When you feel pressured. We do know that many cats and dogs are euthanized every day, however, if you are looking for one for your home, don't be swayed by the threat of "this one will die if you don't adopt today." There are many animals on death row, and many more in no-kill shelters. The one you choose is the life you save.

When you are doing it to impress someone else. Some people will adopt because they believe it will make them appear to be a caring person, when in actuality, the animals is not really getting the love they deserve at home.

Remember that adopting a cat or dog is a lifetime commitment. Adopt for the right reasons.

Shannon was looking for a designer dog that would look good on the end of a leash. She visited all the boutique dog breeders looking for the one that would make her look good.
One day a friend invited her to visit a local shelter. The dog that caught her eye and then her heart is now the best accessory in her life, and they do look good together.

Adoption Websites

Some of the websites I have found helpful are:
www.petfinder.com,
www.adoptapet.com
www.pets911.com.

Also, if there is a particular breed you are interested in, there usually is a rescue organization for that particular breed.

I do not have personal experience with any of these following rescues, however this list came by way of recommendations from friends who have used them:

Dogs:
Boston Terriers: www.bostonbuddies.org
Italian Greyhounds: www.italiangreyhound.org
Collies: www.collie.org
Pugs: www.pugdogrescue.com
Golden Retriever http://adopt-a-golden-retriever.adoptapet.com
Miniature Schnauzers www.schnauzerrescue.net
Standard Poodle http://www.standardpoodlesusa.com/poodle-rescue.html

Bichon Frise
http://www.rescueinfocenter.com/index.php?c=Bichon+Frise
Pomeranian Rescue http://www.secondchancepoms.org
Chow Dog rescue http://www.chowdog.com
Yorkshire Terriers http://www.saveayorkierescue.org/

Cats:
Save a Cat http://www.saveacat.org
Every cat counts http://www.everycatcounts.info
Purebred Cat Breed Rescue http://purebredcats.org

I have personal experience with Pet Orphans in Southern California which is where I first met Tigger:
www.petorphans.org

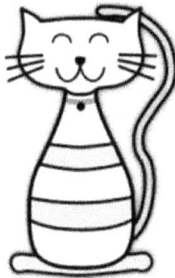

"Animals have these advantages over man:
they never hear the clock strike,
they die without any idea of death,
they have no theologians to instruct them,
their last moments are not disturbed by unwelcome
and unpleasant ceremonies,
their funerals cost them nothing,
and no one starts lawsuits over their wills."

~ Voltaire

CLOSING

Cats and dogs are not toys. They are not accessories to be discarded at the change of fashion. They are wonderful loving hearts that will love you for their lifetime. They count on your to teach them, protect them and love them for your lifetime as well.

This book is only the beginning. There are so many more awesome stories where we can learn from our animal companions and each other. We welcome your stories. Visit the website www.stressout-book.com to submit your story. Perhaps you'll read it in a future edition and your words can helps someone else.

ABOUT THE AUTHORS & CONTRIBUTORS

Sumner M. Davenport
Primary Author, Publisher

Sumner Davenport is a Solutions Consultant, a best-selling author, publisher, sought after public speaker and she is quoted often. One of Sumner's quotes was voted by an independent group to be included in the Top 10 Healthy Thoughts of 2007. (*Struggle ends where commitment begins*). As a self-worth advocate and a proponent of self-investment rather than self-improvement, Sumner trademarked the phrase " *The investments we make in ourselves always deliver the most profitable returns.*"

She is author and co-author of several books including, Solving the Entrepreneur Puzzle, It Works with Simple Keys, Stress Out, Show stress who's the boss™; Stress Out for Cats, Dogs & their People, A Difference a Day Makes and more. In many of her books, Sumner brings together co-authors, professionals, stories & testimonials to provide a variety of solutions for the reader. A portion of the proceeds from all her books benefit selected charities.

As a publisher, Sumner works with emerging authors to assist them in achieving their goals being a published author and having their books reach their target market. Sumner also strives for all of her client's books to be suitable for charity fundraising, corporate promotions and educational purposes.

Among her awards she has been acknowledged by The Los Angeles Superior Court for her "Outstanding Service to Children", Southern California Small Business Owners as Entrepreneur of the Year; the Lioness Club for her "Examples in Leadership"; Networker of the Year by Women's Referral Service where she also held the volunteer position as president of the Westlake/Thousand Oaks Chapter and AVProz for her participation as board member.

She can be reached www.SumnerDavenport.com; Sumner@SumnerDavenport.com
Facebook Business Page:
http://facebook.dj/sumner.davenport

Janine Allen

Janine Allen is Rescue Me Dog's professional dog trainer. Janine's passion is working with people and their dogs. She provides demonstrations for those who have adopted shelter dogs, lends email support to adopted dog owners that need information beyond the website's Training Support Pages; and aids shelter staff and volunteers in understanding dog behavior to increase their adoptability. Janine is the original author of "I Rescued a Human Today". It is published in this book with her full permission. She can be reached through www.rescuemedog.org

Ellen "Ellie" Bishop

Ellie Bishop began her career as a veterinarian technician in an animal shelter located in Charleston, South Carolina. She began by taking her daughter to the local shelter to volunteer. During the first few weeks, she would play with dogs, scratch kittens' ears, and help the staff with extra requests they might have. This shelter was old, had many out building trailers for additional space, and was making due the best they could with what they had. The staff was incredibly compassionate, always keeping the animals' best interest at the core of what they were doing. After a few weeks, the shelter manager asked her to join the staff. This began her journey into the shelter world of animal care.

Some of the animals in her poems are now her personal companions, others have gone on to the Rainbow Bridge, and yet others have found 'furrever' loving homes. As a certified euthanasia technician, it was her unfortunate, yet necessary job to ensure those who were put to sleep were given the compassion and gentle touch they deserved when leaving this earth. She has spent many nights shedding tears over those that she could not help. To provide more understanding of each animal in her poems, she has included the short story about them.

Ellie recently attended the Culinary Institute of Charleston and is now a full time chef. She continues to spend volunteer time helping animals in need. To contact Ellie, please visit http://stressoutforcatsanddogs.com

🐾 Dr. Kim Bloomer

Dr. Kim, as she is affectionately known, is a veterinary naturopath. She also is the host and creator of Animal Talk Naturally Radio show which she hosts together with her like-minded colleague and friend, Dr. Jeannie Thomason. She is also a proficient blogger and writer on natural pet health. Dr. Kim is also co-author of the book Whole Health for Happy Dogs and author of the book Animals Taught Me That. Dr. Kim's articles have been featured in various publications such as Animal Wellness Magazine, Natural Horse Magazine, and Dogs...Naturally Magazine. She is adjunct professor with Kingdom College of Natural Health. Dr. Kim lives with her husband of many years. Visit her website at http://www.AspenbloomPetCare.com

❧ Victoria Loveland-Coen

Victoria Loveland-Coen is an inspirational speaker, the author of two books, Manifesting Your Desires, and The Baby Bonding Book; a mother-of-twins, and Aurora's best friend. Her blog, The Gratitude Experiment (www.gratitudexp.com) promotes and supports the practice of "proactive" gratitude as an effective method for transforming our lives...and the world. Her Gratitude Experiment page is quickly becoming a favorite destination for thousands on Facebook. (http://www.facebook.com/pages/The-Gratitude-Experiment/308476274124)

❧ Tammy Lawrence-Cymbalisty

Tammy Lawrence-Cymbalisty is the owner/operator of TLC Services. She holds many certifications including; Certified Yoga teacher, Reiki Master/teacher and Clinical Hypnotherapist. You can find out more about Tammy on her website at http://www.reikiandyoga.com

❧ Dina Discola

After her experience with purchasing a dog, Dina became a volunteer for a no-kill animal shelter called New Leash on Life (NLOL.org) and has educated herself on how important it is to rescue or foster. She also earned the status of Certified Handler in a therapy program called Lend a Paw (LAP). Dina consistently supports animal rescue causes. She adopted Charlie Brown who she talks about in "A Charlie Brown Christmas" from BostonBuddies.com. Dina can be seen frequently at fundraising events with her dogs. In 2012 she and Charlie raised funds and attention for "Strutt Your Mutt" and the Best Friends Animal Society. To contact Dina please visit http://stressoutforcatsanddogs.com

🐾 Lynda Fishman

Lynda Fishman is a trained clinical social worker who has spent over twenty years as a camp director. In the early 90s, Lynda was one of the first camp directors in the Toronto area to incorporate children with special needs into mainstream camp life. Lynda has devoted a lifetime to organized camping and is passionate about the positive role of camping in a person's life. Lynda is a motivational and inspirational speaker and facilitator. She has published articles and training manuals on leadership, teamwork, bullying, trust, childhood health and wellness, communication and customer service. Lynda and her husband Barry have three grown children, and the whole family is heavily involved in supporting children dealing with tragedy, cancer or other life-threatening diseases, fund-raising and charity events. To learn more about Lynda visit her website: http://repairingrainbows.com

🐾 Eileen Gould

Eileen Gould is a licensed General Contractor, Certified Interior Designer, Speaker, Stager, and Winner of the HGTV, Designer Challenge. She can be reached through her website: http://www.lifestylesdesign.com

🐾 Sue Heldenbrand

Sue Heldenbrand received her certification as a Healing Touch practitioner in 2002. She is also a Certified Integrated Energy Therapy Practitioner, a Reiki Practitioner, and a Quantum Touch Practitioner. She uses energy-based therapies for trauma release work with success for people suffering with PTSD or for anyone who has had a traumatic experience in their lives. Following Hurricanes Katrina and Rita, which devastated areas nearby, Sue worked with Volunteers of America as part of the La. Spirit Disaster Relief Team providing stress management and trauma release work with those involved with the victims of these hurricanes.

She has been a guest speaker for numerous organizations. She has written articles on energy work for alternative and complementary newsletters and online publications. She has developed material and has been a trainer for education classes for child care, stress management seminars and subtle body energy workshops.

To learn more about Sue visit her website: http://www.synergisticcenter.com

Sally Shields

Sally Shields is an award-winning pianist, composer, speaker, author and radio personality. A frequent contributor to various magazines, Shields has been featured in Star Magazine, Obvious, My Day, Girlfriends, For the Bride and many others. Endorsed by Dr. Laura Schlessinger and Martha Stewart, she has appeared on Fox & Friends, Rachel Ray, Tyra and the Daily Buzz with her bestseller, *The Daughter-In-Law Rules!* A marketing coach at Outskirts Press, she has also penned, *Publicity Secrets Revealed: What Every PR Firm Doesn't Want you to Know* and *The CollaboratorRules: 101 Surefire Ways to Stay Friends with Your Co-Author!* Her latest tome: *Naturally Thin or Discipline? Insider Secrets of the Super-Slim!* Was released in 2011. Shields lives in New York City with her husband and two children. For more information, please visit: www.sallyshields.com

Dr. Joy Vanderbeck

Dr. Joy Vanderbeck, Ph.D. C.Ht. is a Life Success Coach, Positive Attitude Trainer, Personal, Professional and Relationship Coach and published author. Beginning her 30th year of coaching and training, Dr. Joy is an active consultant, specializing in positive thinking, communication skills, and personal motivation.

In addition to her private practice as a Life Success Coach, Dr. Joy has presented numerous programs to organizations and companies, including Dallas Business Journal, Data Return Corporation, Ebby Halliday REAL-TORS, Re/Max, churches, Rotary, Lions and Kiwanis clubs. She has also conducted classes for Realtors. Mademoiselle Magazine featured Dr. Joy in an article titled, *"Are you too Trusting?"*

Dr. Joy graces her clients, and audiences with an innovative approach for life success, creating an atmosphere in which participants feel enthusiasm to excel.

You can reach her through her website: www.joyv.com or by e-mail: joyv@joyv.com

Additional Contributors

Sharone Ray -" Dog Parks"
Bernard J. (Last name withheld by request) - "My Wife's Cat"
Marcia Klark - "If I knew Then What I Know Now"
Katie W. (Last name withheld by request)- "Only My Dog"
Leslie May - "The Message in Poop"
Mike Branson - "To Leash or Not to Leash"
Cindy S. (Last name withheld by request) - "Car Ride"

"No amount of time can erase the memory of a good cat, and no amount of masking tape can ever totally remove his fur from your couch."

- Leo Dworken

Quote References

Cleveland Amory
was an American author who devoted his life to promoting animal rights. He was perhaps best known for his books about his cat, named Polar Bear, whom he saved from the Manhattan streets on Christmas Eve 1977. The executive director of the Humane Society of the United States described Amory as "the founding father of the modern animal protection movement."

Lauren Bacall
 is an American film and stage actress and model

Dave Barry
is a Pulitzer Prize-winning American author and columnist, who wrote a nationally syndicated humor column for The Miami Herald from 1983 to 2005. He has also written numerous books of humor and parody, as well as comedic novels.

Martin Buber
was an Austrian-born Israeli philosopher

Henry Ward Beecher
was a prominent Congregationalist clergyman, social reformer, abolitionist, and speaker in the mid to late 19th century.

Josh Billings
was the pen name of 19th century American humorist Henry Wheeler Shaw.

Samuel Butler
was an iconoclastic Victorian-era English author.

Roger A. Caras
was an American wildlife photographer, writer, wildlife preservationist and television personality.

Jules Champfleury
was a French art critic and novelist, a prominent supporter of the Realist movement in painting and fiction.

Jean Cousteau
is a French explorer, environmentalist, educator, and film producer.

Leonardo da Vinci
was an Italian Renaissance polymath: painter, sculptor, architect, musician, scientist, mathematician, engineer, inventor, anatomist, geologist, cartographer, botanist, and writer.

Sir Arthur Conan Doyle
was a Scottish physician and writer.

Bill Dana
is an American comedian, actor and screenwriter.

Jim Davis
is an American cartoonist, best known as the creator of the comic strip Garfield.

Ralph Waldo Emerson
was an American essayist, lecturer, and poet,

George Eliot
was the pen name of Mary Anne Evans an English novelist, journalist and translator, and one of the leading writers of the Victorian era.

Anatole France
was a French poet, journalist, and novelist.

Sigmund Freud
was an Austrian neurologist and Founder of psychoanalysis.

Mahatma Gandhi
was the preeminent leader of Indian nationalism in British-ruled India.

Robert A. Heinlein
was an American science fiction writer.

Ernest Hemingway
was an American novelist and short-story writer. He won the Nobel Prize for Literature in 1954.

James Herriot
was the pen name of James Alfred Wight, OBE, FRCVS, a British veterinary surgeon and writer.

Hippocrates
was an ancient Greek physician of the Age of Pericles.

Edward Hoagland
is an author best known for his nature and travel writing

Joseph Wood Krutch
was an American writer, critic, and naturalist.

Wendy Liebman
is an American stand-up comedian.

Groucho Marx
was an American comedian and film and television star. He is known as a master of quick wit and widely considered one of the best comedians of the modern era.

John Muir
was a Scottish-born American naturalist, author, and early advocate of preservation of wilderness in the United States.

Gilda Radner
was an American comedian and actress, best known as one of the original cast members of the NBC sketch comedy show Saturday Night Live.

Jerry Seinfeld
is an American stand-up comedian, actor, writer, and television/film producer.

Robert Southey
was an English poet of the Romantic school, one of the so-called "Lake Poets", and Poet Laureate for 30 years

Robert Louis Stevenson
was a Scottish novelist, poet, essayist, and travel writer.

Mark Twain
the pen name of Samuel Langhorne Clemens, was an American author and humorist.

Anne Tyler
is a Pulitzer Prize-winning American novelist.

Jules Verne
was a French author who pioneered the science fiction genre.

Voltaire
was the nom de plume of François-Marie Aroue, a French Enlightenment writer, historian and philosopher famous for his wit and for his advocacy of civil liberties.

QUOTE REFERENCES

Thornton Wilder
was an American playwright and novelist. He won three Pulitzer Prizes.

Ben Ames Williams
was an accomplished American novelist and short story writer.

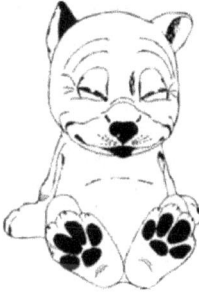

References

1.) http://www1.umn.edu/news/features/2008f/UR_176613_REGION1.html

2.) www.arthritis.org/pet-stretch.php

3) UK study available on Stress Out for Cats, Dogs & their People website

4.) Abstract available on Stress Out for Cats, Dogs & their people website

5.) http://www.usfca.edu/law/news/dogtherapy

6.) http://www.emeraldinsight.com/journals.htm?issn=1753-8351&volume=5&issue=1&articleid=17024849&show=abstract&PHPSESSID=543ve0ndjt4etv931u0v8i2p81)

7.) http://www.cmp.wisc.edu/faculty/bio.php?name=jgern

8.) http://consensus.nih.gov/1987/1987HealthBenefitsPetsta003html.htm

9.) http://www.webmd.com/hypertension-high-blood-pressure/guide/5-ways-pets-improve-your-health?page=2

10.) http://www1.umn.edu/news/features/2008f/UR_176613_REGION1.html

11.) http://rechai.missouri.edu

12.) http://healthypets.mercola.com/sites/healthypets/archive/2011/02/17/dangers-of-early-pet-spaying-or-neutering.aspx

13.) http://www.aspca.org/pet-care/spayneuter and http://www.spayusa.org

14.) http://actorsandothers.com/bettys_bucks_for_balls.html

15.) http://www.aspca.org/pet-care/pet-care-tips/how-to-remove-a-tick-from-your-pet.aspx

16.) http://med.stanford.edu/news_releases/2005/july/hot-cars.htm

17.) Study available on Stress Out for Cats, Dogs & their people website

18.) http://www.adoa.org/state/colorado/3956-larimer-county-co-case-of-a-trainer-who-beat-his-own-dog-could-lead-to-regulations-for-dog-trainers

19.) http://www.azcentral.com/arizonarepublic/local/articles/2012/08/31/20120831animal-cruelty-laws-phoenix-scrutiny.html

20.) http://www.azleg.gov//FormatDocument.asp?inDoc=/legtext/50leg/2r/bills/hb2310p.htm&Session_ID=107

21.) http://www.adoa.org/state/illinois/3151-illinois-pet-history-disclosure-law-goes-into-effect

22.) http://www.mainelegislature.org/legis/statutes/7/title7sec4152.html

QUOTE REFERENCES

23.) http://www.dailynews.com/news/ci_21367668/l-panel-backs-ban-some-pet-sales
24.) http://www.cga.ct.gov/asp/cgabillstatus/cgabillstatus.asp?selBillType=Bill&bill_num=5409&which_year=2012&SUBMIT1.x=0&SUBMIT1.y=0

Public Domain clipart thanks to http://www.pdclipart.org , http://www.catclipart.net, and openclipart.org

www.ingramcontent.com/pod-product-compliance
Lightning Source LLC
Chambersburg PA
CBHW072114270326
41931CB00010B/1557